HOMEOPATHY – GIFT OF A GRACIOUS GOD

by

Deirdre Kelleher McNamara

Completed on the Feast of St. Luke, Patron of of Physicians 2024

Part one completed on October 4, 2024 – St Francis of Assisi

Contact: deirdresbooks@proton.me

Editor: Mr. Peter McNamara, B.A

Inspiration: Mr. Niccolo McNamara

Media Consultant: Ms. A McNamara

With love and appreciation to my dear patients and to those who have supported me during political adverse and trying times.

Especially in this age of the death cult of THANATOS.

God bless you one and all.

This book may be controversial, so I will reserve your names, for now, especially my MD associates, but you are in my heart and prayers.

I will thank you publicly when it is safe – on your behalf – to so do.

In tribute to the late John Vecchione, M.D., Medical Director of Goldwater Memorial Hospital who opened the doors to Homeopathy for the greater benefit of our patients - after years of corruption and pharmaceutical directed closure.

RIP John – Jesus said "Whatever you do to the least of my people, that you do unto Me!" You risked your career for the sickest of the sick –now may the Lord reward you!

Introduction:

And God said to Moses – "Let Likes Cure Likes!!!"

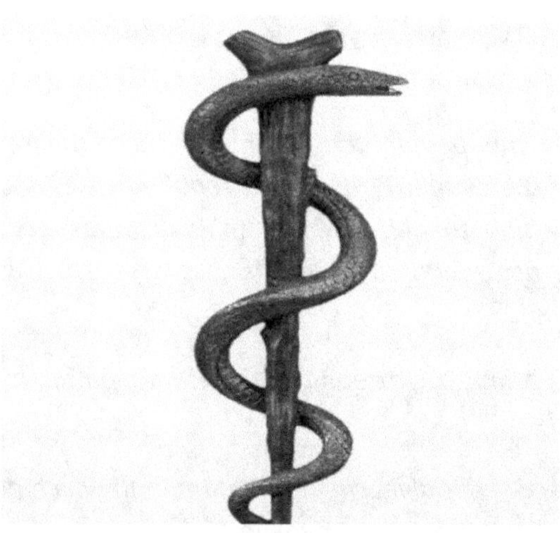

And those who looked upon the snake were cured of the effects of the snake bite! Like Cures Like – the founding principle of Homeopathy!!! From Hippocrates to Hahnemann.

The dynamised, micro-diluted, non-material "ethers" or "images" of our thoroughly investigated remedies be they derived from benign herbs, mysterious minerals or venomous venoms are analogous to the image of the snake.

And just as powerful. As the Hand of God is apparent in the discovery of quinine by St Martin de Porres, and its transport to Europe by Jesuit Missionaries. And its description by the great Dr. Samuel Hahnemann as: "The Gift of a Gracious God!"

And so it was – to me as a bedridden teen, and so it is to those who can find an *authentic* Homeopath and so it will be...*as long as life endures!*

Because if it is of God it will endure. And so it has!

FIRST RULE OF PRESCRIBING: THE LAW OF SIMILARS... Let "alikes cure alikes..."[1]

Salvation – around 1400 B.C., Moses used the bronze serpent on a rod to save his people from snakes sent by God as punishment. Whenever anyone was bitten by a snake and looked at the bronze serpent, he lived.

Nephi tells the people that many of the Israelites perished because of the simplicity and faith required i.e., "and the labor which they had to perform was to look; and because of the simpleness of the way, or the easiness of it, there were many who perished."[2]

One of the prime frustrations of the Homeopath. It's too easy for the patient.

There is a scent of Calvinism in the manner in which patients too readily accept the punitive measures of Allopathy – watch "Doc Martin" for example – and mistrust the inexorably investigated gentle powers of the Homeopath's extraordinary Repertory.

One dose of the perfectly, correctly prescribed "similar" or remedy, dissolved sub lingua, no food or drink for thirty minutes prior or following[3] is "too simple," "too easy" for many, especially those in the pHarma professions who consult us or those who have undergone every arduous procedure required by the Faucis and Rockefeller AMAs directing "health care" in the USA and Europe's Fourth Reich aka the EU!

---

[1] In UK English "Let likes cure likes." US English is more specific, less "flexible" in recognition of the polycultural communities once unique to the USA.

[2] Wikipedia "Nehushtan"

[3] Acute and emergency conditions excepted. Water allowed immediately prior to remedy intake but not for 20 mins after – the limitations increase to one hour before and prior for higher potencies.

Basic comparisons between *Harma Medicine and established, effective alternatives.

Pharma Med	Acupuncture HOMEOPATHY	Herbalism Chinese Herbs
Simplistic	Complex Complex	Simplistic Complex
3rd leading cause of death	Can impair or harm Restorative, never harms	Can be toxic Can be toxic
Suppressive	Curative CURATIVE	Curative or helpful c Helpful
Abuses genetic	Improves genetics Corrects hereditary ills	Helpful Helpful
Abortifacient	Can harm pre-natal baby 100% safe during pregnancy	Abortifacient Abortifacient
One size fits all	Patient specific Precise, specific	Broad range Patient specific
Req. constant review	Range of skills Req. deep skills	Req. knowledge Req. knowledge
Side effects	Twinge on needle insertion NO SIDE EFFECTS	Possible side fx Possible side fx
Controlled x Pharma	Proven rules Law of Similars	Now Pharma Doctrine of Similars
Test tube invention	Chinese monks RC monks, priests, doctors	Catholic monks Chinese monks
Lab tests galore	Pulse diagnoses Intense anamnesis	Observation Obs n evaluation

Dr. Diamond: "Orthodox Medicine is hard to learn but easy to practice. Chinese Herbals–easy to learn, hard to practice. Homeopathy–hard to learn, hardest to practice!

Dr. Murray: "I can see five patients in the time it takes you to see one." Authentic Homeopath: "but ours recover – yours stay on the tablets!!!"

Foreword

HOMEOPATHY – GIFT OF A GRACIOUS GOD!

To a Catholic Editor

I was glad to see dear Archbishop Mansell's name on your page. I was not impressed with a previous HLI (Ireland) speaker.

I hope that you are clear about fighting evil, and not just being a 'shill' for Big Pharma, aka the medicine of Mammon. Happily, your list of lectures suggests the former.

As you may surmise from the front cover, I am a Doctor of Homeopathy, a thoroughly researched and documented therapeutic protocol which has withstood two centuries of persecution and informed most major developments in 'Old School' medicine, as well as warning about the dangers of excess antibiotics and mass vaccinations.

My education was fast tracked. At the age of nine, English educational authorities proved that I had the literacy equivalent of an Oxbridge graduate in literature.

I spent 43, 44 days at school in my Sophomore and Senior years, and still maxed four Math papers, including Calculus, in the Irish Leaving Cert.

I was the "jet propelled" pupil of my piano teacher and winner of multiple awards in Gaelic after studying for only three months, directly off the boat from the New Forest, Hampshire, England.

At 12 years of age I was an *ex officio,* unpaid remedial teacher to 14 year old girls who were kept back.

I have translated scientific documents from Russian at the age of 15, after a few months study of the language, and legal documents from Portugese after no study whatsoever.

"Although you have no training in theory or harmony we still think you are the one most likely to succeed" said the kindly late head of the Julliard Extension School of Composition.

All the grants went to DEI, even then.

Milton Babbitt former Director of ASCAP recommended that I apply for a grant from ASCAP. I submitted my list of Hymns and Masses and was summarily refused. Milton had reassured me that there would be no religious discrimination there. I did not complain to him, as he was so kind. A mistake on my part.

I was too advanced for the Physics in my High School /Secondary School and was coached privately by Professor Gregg of Trinity College.

Despite Boiron's disastrous policy of mass distribution of Homeopathic remedies to be "prescribed" by Health Food Store clerks, Homeopathy is not a faffy hit or miss one symptom fits all protocol.

Yes, one obscure symptom can be a deciding factor in remedy selection or prescription but it must concur with the *totality of the other symptoms.*

And to misquote Shakespeare for a moment; "Symptoms come not in single spies, but in battalions!"

The Homeopath takes on those "battalions" – the totality of symptoms, "delighting" in the "peculiar" symptoms, often the brightest signpost to a precise prescription and rapid cure!

So, yes, we have something far superior to offer. Far superior.

Gamaliel Principle: "If it is from God, it will prevail."

CHAPTER ONE - Gamaliel - Homeopathy prevails!

Homeopathy prevails despite a tsunami of hostility, disinformation and unfounded assaults from associates of the Pharmaceutical industry.

Those strategies in and of themselves require an entire book! They include suppression of evidence; they include "casual" but well sponsored denigrations of Homeopathy in entertainment, e.g. Dr. Kildare, Little House on the Prairie and more recently, Doc Martin. In each and every series, Homeopathy is misrepresented and denigrated.

Doc Martin – in desperate need of ... a Homeopath! I am grateful for the series' expose of the limitations of pHARMakopeia.

More recently, well, around the turn of the last century, strategies become more subtle. Unable to suppress us, they funded glossy "Health care" magazines and articles, lumping us in with traditional, botanical, grandma's kitchen remedies, etc., all which have merit.

However, they are not capable of the deep and precise *curative* work of Homeopathy. By *curative* I mean the elimination of the cause of recurrent symptoms.

Over the last two, three decades, I have noticed the theft and plagiary of language, of our terminology...

The AMA scoffers now promote nutritional awareness, exercise, i.e., fitness, and even the occasional herb or tea...something that can be oriented toward mass sales, all under the heading "Good health."

Some of this is excellent. After all, Doctor Samuel Hahnemann is the father of *Nutrition, Hygiene and recommendations of fresh air, exercise and limited stress.*

*In addition to the creation of an extraordinary new protocol best described as **sub-molecular medicine!***

It won't take long for the sociopathic scoffers in pHARMa medicine to adopt the term "molecular medicine." In fact I believe they already tried purloining that term.

For the materialists scoffing as they read, thinking that there is no material substance other than the "host" *saccarum lactis,* did any ever try to, say, "weigh" oxygen or question the splitting of the atom to generate nuclear **energy...?** [4]

Now, Dr. Samuel Hahnemann developed the extraordinary process of dilution-dynamisation. This process of dynamisation at each stage of dilution releases the exquisite powers of the Homeopathic "remedy," or, more precisely, *"potential,"* because the remedy must *resonate* with the totality of symptoms experienced by the patient, or be of little help, especially in acute cases.

When the "potential" resonates, it is extraordinarily powerful. Gentle, as in no side effects, but powerful.

Freud, Semmelweis, Pasteur were two of his "plagiarists" as was the tragic Edward Jenner the father of death by vaccination – his first victim being his poor son.

Re Hygiene, in Hahnemann's time surgeons would wipe their hands on their outer garments. The more filthy and encrusted the garment, the greater the prestige of the surgeon!

Hahnemann promoted *asepsis, that is, cleanliness.*

The "wannabes" who followed him then came up with *antisepsis.*

---

[4] https://www.energy.gov/ne/articles/fission-and-fusion-what-difference

Hospitals in England were very clean notwithstanding the shared bathrooms of the poor, and they were disinfected with carbolic soap, which, according to some medical historians, were associated with recurrent infections.

I don't have a reference for that. I read copiously, and friends of the pharmaceutical industry made my life unmanageable for many years.

Records often had to be scrapped.

I still managed, thank God, to reach many patients and relieve their suffering. But some were unable to reach me, and passed to the Lord.

Historically, however, before these protocols had a terminology, honey, wine, herbs were used for cleansing and healing and were often, understandably, **effective.**

Homeopathy, on the other hand, is highly individualised, demanding great skill and vital for numbers of "incurable" conditions.

The doctor attached to Knock Shrine, who tried to purloin my Hep C patients as "proof of Knock Miracles" mocked me to my face, saying: "I can see 4, or 5 patients in the time it takes you to see one.

"But mine recover. Yours stay on "the tablets."" His face contorted in rage.

That brief, cold but civil phone conversation was then re-written by his secretary, not present at the time as "Dr McNamara was shouting and hollering in the surgery."

This disinformation and slanderous "specialist" was in a General Practitioner's surgery on the grounds of a celebrated Shrine in Ireland.

This is just one of many such similar incidences around the world – not with my patients, but from persons associated with the Pharmaceutical Industry, or who want a monopoly on suffering!

The same GP was called by the Sacristan of Knock Shrine to attend to a young man who had a seizure inside the Church.

The GP arrived inebriated with the Gardai , ie, "police" and, instead of referring the young men to hospital, claimed that he did not know he had a seizure because he didn't witness it, and ordered the Gardai to arrest the young man.

No grounds for arrest unless they would count seeking safety in the Church as "trespassing."

The GP in question was regularly seen sporting a black eye, which was reputed to be the result of bar fights. However, since I've been the subject of the Knock disinfo machine, and this is logical analysis rather than eye-witness to the possible fights, I'll give him the benefit of the doubt.

For the record, I'm not in competition with God for miracles, but I will uphold the work of authentic Homeopathy, because that saves lives.

On the contrary, I try to limit the need for Divine Intervention, help with the "workload" so to speak, leaving the harshest and most heartbreaking cases for Him.

St Pio says "Don't limit God." This is not "limiting" God but clearing the path for His limitless interventions where genuinely needed, when prior iatrogenic or traumatic "interventions" leave little for our gentle but powerful treatments to work with.

***

CHAPTER TWO - God vs Mammon

Homeopathy is patient friendly but demands great dedication and concentration from the practitioner. We must compare and contrast hundreds, if not thousands of symptoms with those kicked up by various gifts of the Creator - plants, venoms, minerals.

It is almost too easy, too simple and uncomplicated for our patients, to the point where I sometimes wonder if I should walk around in long robes and carry a gong...tapping out mysterious rhythms by a gurgling fountain and charge accordingly!

Watch the chartered jets land nearby!!!!

And yes, a good Homeopath is worth a "King's Ransom," but the "job satisfaction" is so high it's almost an end unto itself – except where the practicalities of survival are concerned.

Hahnemann and the founding fathers of Homeopathy used to treat the rich, charge appropriately, then treat the poor, pro bono.

Meanwhile, back to the "my sister's a nurse and *she* says..."

Or "my doktah says I'm doing really well, but to go back on the pills just in case..." which pills had merely suppressed symptoms for forty years, while the patient's condition and systems deteriorated!

Or the one I fear the most – "the social worker said I had to take him (a child) back to the GP and put him back on the seizure medication."

And my sweet patient goes back down the slippery slope.

In one case, a monk with severe allergies was allowed to consult me. The allergy medications cost $1,000.00 every week. After one week of Homeopathic treatment, his symptoms *completely disappeared.*

The *Abbot* insisted that he resume the asthma medications *against my strongest caution.*

The rebound was predictably intense; not against the external allergens, but against the allergens in the needle that he was forced to take.

The Abbot then insisted he leave the Monastery.

I didn't expect "Papal Honors," so to speak, but a thank you and invitation to lunch would be nice. And an *oath to never sabotage my treatments again!*

Right now, where manners are concerned, the SJs are ahead of the OSBs!

Two other monastic patients were allowed to consult with me, then quickly removed from my care in a most frustrating and obnoxious manner, once their status showed significant improvement.

The monk in charge of the infirmary was a giant of a man, not too fond of women, and strangely possessive of his patients.

They seemed afraid of him.

One died, a sweet and brilliant priest and religious, sitting outside the Chapel door on Easter Sunday, waiting for his brother monks to pull him up the steps. He was a kind and gentle man, very brilliant, from a German family.

He would speak in German to me, and I would understand most of it and reply in my limited German. He didn't seem to mind, and was just happy to express himself in the language of his people. Very sweet priest, RIP.

Meanwhile the other monks were inside the main refectory across the Plaza, enjoying Easter celebrations. In his frustration he tried to wheel his chair up onto terra firma and fell, sustaining a serious head injury and died soon after.

I hope that there was an autopsy.

Two more elderly monks were in an orthodox hospital, seemingly stable, articulate and fed up!

My last patient of that order was a brilliant man; writer, philosopher, theologian and the former Dean of Religion and Philosophy.

He wrote long, involved, autobiographical poems, and while in manageable health, stayed in for "three hots and a cot," as he did not feel that he could live alone.

He was falsely accused of improper conduct with a young female student. His accuser was a lecturer in his faculty'- the crypto-moslem who coveted his position and was, himself, reported to be involved with a young student.

The accuser was certainly close to a moslem tv celebrity, notorious for demonstrating and promoting cannibalism on his show. The accuser tried to persuade the Abbot to allow the cannibal to conduct a seminar. At least that was denied!

The accuser was also encouraging young, male, students to engage in archaeological research in Qumran, Israel, source of the Dead Sea Scrolls.

In recent years, Qumran became notorious for a secondary, non-scholarly aspect: its mostly male "social" life.

I am not a witness to this, if it is true, thank God, but sources appeared credible, accompanied either by grimace or smirk.

The Abbot ordered the calumniated monk to step down and away from public life. That broke something in him, will to live perhaps.

I have wondered from time to time if the Abbot intended to sell the monastery which was attached to a University, at that time under "courtship" by a moslem cannibal and the crypto moslem Associate Dean who had falsely accused his superior of misconduct with a young female student.

The Abbot took the word of the moslem over his own ordained priest and suspended the Dean. Such accusations are very difficult to shake even when the falsely accused party is - exonerated, and the priest was never reinstated.

The gentle slopes, woods and trees surrounding the property would have made an ideal jihadi training ground, and the student dorms were a stone's throw from the Lewis McChord Joint AF base.[5]

Injustice is hard to bear, and, frankly, having had to dodge a "legion" of "Weinsteins" in my literary, dramatic and academic years, I feel obliged to verify that I experienced and sensed nothing "creepy" in this erudite and kindly monk.

His poetry is quite beautiful, with many historical references.

Perhaps one day his poems will be published and celebrated.

If our Church were more invested in promoting Catholic Culture and less in "fish fries" we might have had a Catholic Nobel Prize winner!

Again, as soon as improvements were manifest, my treatments were discontinued by order of the Abbot in collusion with the

---

[5] https://home.army.mil/lewis-mcchord/

woman who kidnapped my grandson and held him in a locked room for forty minutes.

She was the wife of the Dean of the far left WA University, "Evergreen" complete with "Red Square" and far left "mondo bizzaro." The Abbot had appointed her as head of their lay associates, so the academic mafioso prevailed in covering up her crime.

Although, as stated previously, his health was quite manageable, he died within a year or two of my departure, if my memory serves me well.

At least he is free, the rude and uncharitable Abbot now replaced, along with an Archbishop of questionable ethics, and the jihadis did not get to buy the beautiful lands and properties, to continue their destruction of "all things and all manner of things" [6]Christian, praise the Lord.

***

---

[6] "all will be well and all manner of things shall be well," famous saying of St Julian of Norwich, anchoress and English Saint.

CHAPTER THREE – The Battle

For those dedicated to the "Relief of Human Suffering"[7] the harassment imposed on the authentic Homeopath is the price we pay for the ability to generate comfort and often complete healing in our beloved patients, and in the insights provided by this system, called by its founder "The Gift of a Gracious God."

Unfortunately, having failed to suppress us, Big Pharma embarked on a campaign in the eighties and nineties to confuse the public, so now I have to battle an array of persons trying to mix in and conflate occultism with this purest of all therapeutic forms. Let me make it very clear:

OCCULTISM HAS NO PLACE IN HOMEOPATHY.

HOMEOPATHY is a precise and gentle science; Samuel Hahnemann is constantly being proven correct, thorough, and even prophetic in his brilliant and logical mind, although constantly plagiarised by "soy-entists" and still not given due credit. I flee from anyone trying, for example, to say "I can find your remedy through your astrological sign…"

That is so insulting to our precise methodologies. Almost as insulting as the "one note" prescriptions promoted by Boiron and Ollois.

On one hand it is wonderful that the remedies are now easily available: On the other it is outrageous that they were not accompanied by major educational endeavours in conveying the awesome, deep and authentic powers of authentic Homeopathy, when practiced correctly.

Sad to say, they may have succumbed to pressure from Fauci's friends at the NIH.

---

[7] "Relief of Human Suffering" is the Foundation of St. Padre Pio's "hospital" on the Gargano mountain of S. Giovanni Rotondo.

Few people know that the "AMA" that is, the American Medical Association was founded for the **suppression** of Homeopathy, not exactly for the maintenance of high Medical Standards.

That was already the "domain" of Rockefeller's *harmaceutical ghouls.

Around the time of the establishment of a major cancer Hospital in the middle of New York City by **London based bankers!!!**

Authentic "Science" is the *study of Creation* and when prayerfully practiced, provides "best use" and guides us as to the purpose of the wonderful elements, vegetations, and animal life gifted as consolation to the great grandchildren of Adam and Eve.

What a succinct exposition of male-female characteristics. "Blokey" Adam, just happy in the garden with his mate, and "ambitious" Eve – has to know everything, tries to take control of the forbidden apple, the one forbidden substance, the fruit of the Tree of Knowledge, leading to disaster.

Like the pHARMacists who take one substance from our "repertory" and abuse it to death, leading to mistrust in our remedies, even though the methods used were anything *except* genuine Homeopathy!

They are even less subtle than +sa+an+!

The serpent is the "liar and father of lies, and a murderer."

Big *harma doesn't just lie. It cheats, dissembles, shadowbans, bribes, funds cute tele series,e.g., Doc Martin, General Hospital, etc., kills even... small creatures, large creatures, even humans.

Big *harma prevents and obstructs Homeopaths from treating even the patients who are beyond and outside their allopathic suppressants.

Suppressive medication can buy time for an exhausted patient and rest for their autologous immune systems to recover, kick in and complete the cure. *If* the symptoms are not too profound, intense, or prolonged and adequate food and fluid is available.

When the medications are nature based and can address both symptoms and *causa radica*.

Humanity and nature co-operated for centuries, occasionally destroying or damaging one another, but there is a subliminal recognition in the human genomic system, the linguistic over-ride, the super consciousness, that "comprehends" and co-operates with the provided plant or creature based meds.

After all the species that survived floods, earthquakes, hurricanes, tornados, volcanic eruptions, violent tectonic abruptions, hailstorms, blizzards, violent electric storms, global warming, global coolings, plagues, drought leading to dehydration-dessication of the earth's mantle, famine, "natural" plagues[8], meteors, etc., must have *something* in common, some natural empathy and compatibility.

Plants do signal their Creator's intentions, in what botanists and herbalists refer to as the *"Doctrine* of Similars."

Ours is the "Law of Similars." A giant leap forward!

CHAPTER FOUR – Herbs vs *harma!

---

[8] Naturally occurring plagues, e.g., bubonic plague, famine induced cholera – e.g., Ireland, vs "plagues" or epidemics directly induced by the flu vaccines of 1918. Bubonic and Cholera were direct consequences of human evils, the blockage of the Mediterrannean trade routes by moslems determined to engage Christians in the slave trade and the abuse of Ireland's resources by Queen Victoria, glutton.

Contemporary Pharmaceuticals are lab based concoctions, alien to humanity...

They are suppressive rather than re-generative. They often address one symptom, but introduce new ones commonly known as "side effects."

Suppression of these require more artificial poly chemicals.

And so the condition deteriorates within, some meds being stored in the liver, others damaging the spleen, intestine, kidneys, etc.

Defiance of the Creator's one command led to expulsion from the Garden of Eden, aka Paradise.

"I'd rather not know," "A little knowledge is a dangerous thing" are mainstay phrases in English colloquia! Applies particularly to Big *harma!

I advise all persons with chronic or 'incurable' illnesses to seek a Homeopath who is AUTHENTIC and Hahnemannian, that is, true to *foundational principles.*

We may not cure all, especially if the patient has already been subject to the *harmacists' destruction of the immune and other vital systems placed by the Divine Creator within the human genome, but I have never met a patient whose status I could not improve. For example...

Even in the case of END STAGE CANCER:

That includes a senior citizen sent "home alone" by her oncologists, with a batch of interferon, to use daily after the bombardments of "radiation" and chemo "therapy" at Memorial Sloan Kettering failed.

She was young and fit for her age, beautiful, former ballerina. I found the diagnosis of Hepatic and Pancreatic Cancer highly questionable. She had none of the irritability and skin discolorations that I encountered in many patients diagnosed with Liver cancer. She did have the gentleness that seems to accompany Pancreatic Cancer, or diagnoses thereof.

Living in a 5th floor walk-up apartment in her condition was cruel. She had no life, no energy, just the interferon and a very staunch friend. Her oncologist agreed to monitor her status if she accepted my care and cancel the interferon.

It took a few weeks, but her life changed dramatically!

And changed for the better!

She returned to work part time, went to theatre, dinner with her friends, etc., and for several years enjoyed an active social life..

Now, not exactly running a marathon, Heaven forbid but enjoying significantly improved health and quality of life.

I call it "death by NY landlord." After 19 days of 90F weather, she appeared so dehydrated – living on the 5th floor apartment with no intercom for, say, food deliveries – that I took the unusual step of contacting her oncologist and asked that she be admitted overnight for re-hydration therapies.

He obliged – and prescribed *copious amounts of Lasix, a powerful diuretic!*

Her condition deteriorated significantly, she was moved to Hospice in the Bronx and she died a few weeks later. Iatrogenic murder!

There is no rationale nor excuse for an Rx of Lasix for a severely dehydrated patient!

That, friends, is the sad side of Homeopathy – sabotage by the criminal element of pHARMa medicine.

Watching the pharmashills destroy our work and being helpless to avoid it.

Watching them coerce vaccinations on children and gouge for every single action, necessary and unnecessary...and

Poison AIDS patients to death... *With antibiotics!!!*

Common factor in the larger AIDS community – chronic, repeat, exotic infections requiring accelerating quantities of antibiotics, each dose destroying the immune system...there is a reason AIDS is called "ACQUIRED Immune Deficiency Syndrome," because it is acquired by prolonged and repeated use of ...

ANTIBIOTICS...

Anti = against

Bio = LIFE

"Well, living organisms," they say.

"Yes, the good ones and the bad ones! The health giving ones and the life destroying ones..."

"Well what else would you have us do...?"

READ MY BOOKS AND GET BACK TO ME.

OH, and no more freebies for the *harmaceutical industry.

I do not expect reciprocity for limiting the toxicity of some of their products, but neither do I expect attempts on my life and forced, perjury based, corruption driven evictions from my homes in the USA, nor vandalism of my home in Ireland...after a smear campaign emanating from the local GP's office.

And yet, that is how they work, even sabotaging their own treatment. Concealing the use of oxycontin while the Homeopath jumps through mental hoops wondering why the patient's recovery is so limited, etc., because relief from suffering means no more oxycontin!

And some would rather have their organs removed than give it up! It is that evil, that addictive.

CHAPTER 5 – "Incurable" Infections

In Knock I "earned" the wrath of the local GP[ii] by CURING not one but *four* recovering addicts of Hepatitis C. within 2,3 months of treatment.

He had proof of the cures, but chose to let people across Ireland die. Shortly after, a whispering campaign started, aided and abetted by HLI's speaker, Johnette Benkovich, ex EWTN, not qualified to speak on anything, imo.

She is alleged to have stated that Homeopathy was "sa+anic," along with other health protocols – none with the power and "authority" of Homeopathy, but most offering helpful, Divinely created or inspired therapeutics, e.g., herbs, minerals, vitamins, beneficial if used correctly and appropriately.

My one reservation is re Reiki, which, as it involves touch and "meditation" may depend on the philosophy and Christian fidelity of the practitioner.

Transdermal absorption is more complex than the absorption of toxins! Energies, "chakras" or meridian lines can also be affected by touch, movement, sound and used for control...

There are other alternatives which are to be avoided, which do have sa*anic origins, and ultimate effects.

It is interesting to watch Obama – nominal U Chicago "professor" use the same hand control movements on Redfield that Meghan Markle uses on Prince Harry.

So many Catholic pundits completely ignore the toxicity, side effects, iatrogenic injury, homicidal intent and consequences of most pharmaceutical products and related procedures, especially abortion, euthanasia, organ theft, vaccinations, most lethally the mRNA bioweapon, reported to have caused the death of 17 milion and idolise the "doktah!"

The true death count is believed to be more to the extent of 33 million humans exterminated, a significant number having organs stolen and no official autopsies allowed.

Significant, however, are the covert autopsies in Italy and the USA. Holes in lungs turned to wet sponges by kidney destroying Remdesivir and / or Midozalam and then the lungs punctured by high pressure oxygen pushed through the vents.

And the Church was silent. Or complicit?

Where were the Johnette Benkovitches, and the Fr Rippengers???

As for Reiki,I know one practitioner - a nun in NY! I don't recommend it, nor any of the New Age practices stated in HLI's publicity, but saw no overt harm. There are huge risks, however, in allowing occultists to touch and hold any part of your person, hand, foot, head, etc.

I do recommend Hatha Yoga - that is, simple stretching and breathing. It is calming and oxygenizing, logical, syntheistic.

Any other form of yoga and you're on your own, as I suspect, many of the extreme forms are antagonistic to the original premise of strengthening the skeleto-muscular system, oxygenating the circulatory systems, and reinforcing and controlling the respiratory system, with overall benefits to central nervous and immune systems. Extremes such as "hot yoga" are attractive to ambitious personalities, being competitive and conducive to rapid weight loss.

They are, however, antithetical to Hatha Yoga, which is quasi Buddhist in its orientation to serenity and acceptance, and consistent with the work of the Creator.

Caution: Said acceptance, however, can then lead to passivity. No "Fire of the Holy Spirit!"

Although Catholic, myself, I respect the search for our Divine Creator which is intrinsic to all genuine religions, albeit bemused by the reluctance of many to acknowledge and embrace Him, and deeply concerned by the willingness of even *educated Christians* to accept on face value the most virulent, criminal and homicidal ideology of all time, possibly excepting the Aztecs, and to invite them en masse into the Christian towns, villages, cities and nations of the world.

Symbols and Sacramentals from our own, Divinely bestowed faith are stolen and twisted and used abominably, *contrary to intent and function, in fact, parody thereof.*

That does not make them Catholic, nor does the abuse of our prayer assists distort or deform our Faith in any way.

So too with the abuse of the profound, Divinely inspired knowledge, science, wisdom and deep research of the early Homeopathists.

Abusing our remedies, avoiding first principles and conflating the term "Homeopathy" with the generic adjective "holistic" does not alter this "Gift of a Gracious God"[9] in any way.

It does, however, dangerously confuse the public.

Like variations on a theme of Christianity?

For example, when Philadelphia based Boericke and Tafel were the primary providers of Homeopathic remedies, used almost exclusively by trained, dedicated, professional Homeopaths, I never heard "We tried Homeopathy but it didn't work."

Not once.

---

[9] "Homeopathy is the Gift of a Gracious God." Samual Hahnemann, Founding Father of Homeopathy. St Martin de Porres is our "grandfather.

Now that remedies are supplied from companies based in countries where Homeopathy is banned, discouraged or put in the control of hopeless, hapless Pharma docs, I hear that frequently.

Takes less than a minute to confirm that Homeopathy was either conflated with Herbalism or that the remedies were used by clueless incompetents, reading "one note" symptoms and dosages from the Blue Tube labels!

Three times a day???

NO!

That's for the allopaths clunky "old school" prescriptions.

CHAPTER 6 – Killing for Profit? Death by Design?

And the world goes... hurray for Doctor False Cheat... IDOLATRY of a small, deranged, homicidal MAN? Now how did Hitler happen?

If the Church says that being an organ donor is an "act of charity," with full knowledge of the fact that Fauci brought the proning- paralysing - organ theft – via induced death by pressurised oxygen pushing techniques from communist china, for the annihilation of the Christian West, and for profiteering motives, then the Church is wrong, wrong, wrong and must make amends!

But was it the Church? Or infiltrators, Judases, corrupt advisers?

If those spox for the Church are ignorant of the methods used, then they are at fault for not keeping up with the techniques used in these vile institutions by these ghoulish surgeons, licensed and determined to kill.

Yes, credit to the physicians of the "Hippocratic Oath era" – who resigned rather than participate in mass genocide.

Those dedicated physician respected by, and known personally to me, graduated before Roe v Wade (1973) and studied and graduated in European Universities where Medicine was still a calling rather than a "get rich quick pharmaslave" – free week-ends in Cancun – lifestyle choice!

And, with the nightmare costs of Medical "education," it takes heroic integrity to ignore the incentives flashing like neon lights at a Casino in Vegas!

The abortion-pushing, pill-dependency promoting *harmaceutical industry is served mostly by amoral "technicians" and protected by politicians, presumably lucrative shareholders, the Silence of our (RC) Church and the willingness of the Catholic Health Care system to comply with the Federal rules and regulations that accompany Federal Funding of schools and hospitals, via Medicaid, Medicare, etc., and the huge dividends enjoyed by share-holders in Big *Harma.

No surprise that three Catholic Hospitals in NY closed by the turn of the 21st Century, possibly under the weight of impending litigation: St. Vincent's, St. Luke's, Cabrini, Bayley Seton, St. Elizabeths, St. Lukes-Roosevelt, Mt Sinai – St Lukes...

Who or what annihilated the Catholic Health Care System?

Compromise?

Heaven help us if their Medical Grads are as deficient as a certain Harvard grad with a BA in World Literature who recognised not one major author, poet, essayist or dramatist from the USA, Europe or South America.

Now with AI and the dearth of the ethos of professional ethics and personal responsibility, remarkably demonstrated by Kimberley Cheatle, former Director of the Secret Service, the absence of any oversight into Elon Mosk's "Neuralink" nor in contesting the ideology of a depraved man, the genocidal enthusiast named Harari, the world is on the brink of potential annihilation. But that's for another book, and more research on the authenticity of reports from "respectable" and "respected" scientific institutions.

Right.

Neuralink? Is the man MAD? Who funds and enables this human –into robot project? Who even allows it to begin? It is THE MOST GENOCIDAL AND DESTRUCTIVE PROJECT SINCE COVID.

Implantation of brain chip??? Really?   And the "great" "protectors of public health" who bully and shadow ban Homeopaths everywhere, stay schtum????

How dare they!

And in whom are they implanted? Who has given consent? Who is aware of the extreme risks of said brain "chips," the *lethality of said chips... as they migrate through the brain, affecting and shutting down one cognitive area after another, finally auto inserting into the circulatory system, and just like the mRNA "clot shot"- directly into the heart!*

Not one of those lab-researched products currently on the markets and pushed at great expense into the arms and mouths of innocents, can equal nor even approach the efficacy of the discoveries of Catholic monastic herbalists, let alone the "Gift of a Gracious God," aka Homeopathy.

Anything *harma claims to do, we have done and continue to do better, and anything that works in their field is either stolen directly from Catholic monks or is purloined from the Homeopaths and distorted. Pharma may place their people in Government agencies, NGOs, Academia; they can bribe, bully or perjure themselves in order to close our hospitals, destroy our records, discourage future practitioners, but ***if it is of God it will prevail.***[10]

---

[10] Prophet-Rabbi Gamaliel, re Jesus.

CHAPTER 7 – The Gift of a Gracious God

Gamaliel was right. Authentic Homeopathy has prevailed, even succeeded incomparably, under the most intense abuse, oppression, even persecution.

Patient on respirator for 16 months in hospital with MRSA, concommitants, etc. One week of Homeopath protocols and he was *free from infection;* two months under Homeopathic care and he was off the vents, a month later, he was wheeling himself around in a wheelchair. Six months later, the paralysed hand was writing, albeit with a slight tremor, which continued to improve.

When I first arrived in the USA, Pharmacists were afraid to talk to us – even though at least one had Victorian lab bottles with the names of our remedies, and some even with the word: "Homeopathy."

Then the execs started to invite us to lunch, with chaperones, in order to "pick out brains," re toxic effects, and find ways in which to compete, never to hire us directly as consultants.

Over two centuries of indisputable proof of efficacy, superior results with the most serious of diseases, with global epidemics, with genetic predispositions, infertility, trauma, etc., and the most deeply researched protocol since time began.

Why? How?

The hand of God guided St Martin de Porres of Peru to the discovery of the Cinchona Bark, aka Quinine. He gave to the Jesuit Missionaries to bring it to Europe where Dr Samuel Hahnemann was inspired to use it to cure is sick friend of cholera by inspiration of his studies of the great Hippocrates.

The remarkable results relative to his "resurrected" friend inspired him to thoroughly research and develop the most amazing therapeutic system, Divinely inspired and light years beyond the purview of " Pharmatech's dangerous and defunct "old school" system.

Elsewhere I mentioned the late, great, Cardinal O'Connor's interest in introducing Homeopathy into the Catholic Health Care System.

My first question – why so long, so late when there was almost two centuries of evidence upholding our claims and the genius of Hahnemann.

Why did the Catholic Health Care system opt into control by pHARMa meds, particularly with their WWII connections to the Third Reich and deep, integrated connectivity to the Hitlerian genocidal stratagem.

Was it to hook into Federal Health Care money, the outrageous overbilling of the Medicare-Medicaid system by the *HARMA industry, that has made trillionaires of Pfizer-GSK, Merck, etc., etc.,ad nauseum?

And is the subsequent closure of so many Catholic Hospitals in NY related to this, or just the soaring demand for "Real Estates" and more apartment buildings subsidised by an increasingly controlling neo communist Federal Government, and it's sa*anic "marriage" to profiteering *harmakopeia… a union which allows private business to experiment, or "trial" their products on helpless patients in NY's State Hospitals.

Against the Homeopath's advice.

As usual!

CHAPTER 8 -COMMANDMENTS *contra* ORGAN DONATION

The "vaccine," the organ theft, the donor racket, abortion, the AZT racket, etc., are NOT the will of God.

How can they be; they are so contra natura, so apposite and opposing to God's benevolent plan for humanity, that they can only be from the dark side. God did not create zombies. He created cogent, intelligent, loving individuals — albeit with independent minds.

I am no theologian, though I sometimes wonder if L***fer's betrayal was so shocking to the Lord that He Created humans in the hope that we would voluntarily choose Him...

However, evil too often ambushes and destroys the human heart.

It is up to HIS creatures, "we the people," to choose to do HIS Will and follow HIS Commandments... only ten — ten succinct laws!

Ten Commandments. Now why are admonitions against idolatry, murder, slander, theft of character, property, spouse, so hard to understand and follow???

The Will of God is *in* those commandments, starting with the First: "I am the Lord Thy God, thou shalt have no God's before me," yet we deify "soyentists" - whose work is nothing more than the STUDY OF CREATION, who cannot **create** so much as a single cell.

We idolatrise the pathogenic, germ breeding, oxygen restricting masks; we fear this photoshopped "dryer ball" i.e., the covid icon, as if it were more powerful than God, the Creator, who doesn't even have to blink to destroy it, if it even existed as originally described!

The Fifth Commandment, that is, "Thou shalt not kill," that is, take human life, by abortion, or any other means such as the death jab, aka the clotshot, the proning-paralysing-push lung destroying pressurised oxygen... what is that if not MURDER? KILLING FOR PROFIT? That's okay then, good for the economy! And the world goes... hurray for Doctor False Cheat... IDOLATRY MAN, and that is NOT the Will of God.

If the Church says that being an organ donor is an "act of charity" with full knowledge of the fact that Fauci brought the proning- paralysing - organ theft — via induced death by pressurised oxygen pushing techniques from communist china, for the annihilation of the Christian West, and for profiteering motives, then the church is wrong, wrong, wrong and must make amends.

If those spokespersons for the Church are ignorant of the methods used in purloining organs from living donors, then they are at fault for not keeping up with the techniques developed and in development in "healthcare" institutions, now licensed and determined to kill.

Yes, credit to the physicians of the "Hippocratic Oath era" — who resigned rather than participate in mass genocide, genocide by torturous cruelty.

The MDs known to, and respected personally by me, graduated before Roe v Wade (1973) and studied and graduated in European Universities where Medicine was still a "calling" rather than a "get rich quick pharmaslave" — free week-ends for Cancun "seminars" — lifestyle choice.

Our protocols may differ, but the dedicated MDs with whom I have worked are definitely worthy of respect and affection. Most resigned rather than participate in the Covid scam at huge personal cost. Better that than blood on their hands.

Now the abortion pushing, pill dependency promoting *harmaceutical industry is served mostly by amoral "technicians" and protected by the Silence of our (RC) Church and the willingness to comply with the Federal rules and regulations that accompany Federal Funding of schools and hospitals, via Medicaid, Medicare, etc., the "slippery slope" of compromise.

No surprise that three Catholic Hospitals in NY closed by the turn of the Century, possibly under the weight of impending litigation: St. Vincent's, St. Luke's, Cabrini, Bayley Seton, St. Elizabeths, St. Lukes-Roosevelt, Mt Sinai – St Lukes...

Who or what annihilated the Catholic Health Care System?

Compromise?

Heaven help us if today's Medical Grads are as defunct as the Harvard grad with a BA in World Literature and who recognised *not one* major author, poet, dramatist from the USA, Europe or South America. NI's Bricklayers are better educated and a delight! As are NI's MDs.

Now with AI and the death of the ethos of personal responsibility, recently and remarkably demonstrated by Kimberley Cheatle, former Director of the Secret Service, the absence of any oversight into Elon Mosk's "Neuralink" nor in contesting the ideology of a depraved man, the genocidal enthusiast named Harari.

Not one of those lab-researched products currently on the markets and pushed at great expense into the arms and mouths of innocents, can equal or even approach the efficacy of the discoveries of Catholic monastic herbalists, let alone the "Gift of a Gracious God," aka Homeopathy.

Over two centuries of indisputable proof of efficacy, superior results with the most serious of diseases, with global epidemics, with genetic predispositions, infertility, trauma, etc., and the most deeply researched protocol since time began.

Why? How?

The hand of God guided St Martin de Porres of Peru to the discovery of the Cinchona Bark, aka Quinine. He gave to the Jesuit Missionaries to bring it to Europe where old school Pharmacist and Physician, Dr Samuel Hahnemann was inspired to use it to cure a sick friend of cholera following the inspiration of his analyses of the insights of the great Greek - Hippocrates.

His friend was dying, fever refusing to resolve to well established herbal decoctions.

Hahnemann noted the similarity of the totality of his friend's symptoms to the effects of over consumption of quinine, at that time relatively new to the West.

Inspired by Hippocrates' "Similia similibus curenter" he *persuaded* his friend to take a few drops and ... *mirabilie Dictu ...* his friend's fever subsided and the road to recovery was well established. And Hahnemann's path to greatness dawned!

The remarkable results relative to his "resurrected" friend inspired him to thoroughly research and develop the most amazing therapeutic system, Divinely inspired and light years beyond the purview of " Pharmatech's dangerous and defunct "old school" system.

The barbarity of contemporary medicine makes the barbarity of the primitives appear benign.

The Collusion of the Judeo Christian Religions is this gross violation of the 5th Commandment given directly to Moses by the Creator is staggering.

The Shepherds are now feeding the wolves.

CHAPTER 9 - ORGAN THEFT aka "harvesting"

"If the person is alive when the organs are retrieved, is it "murder?"

Yes, "Patrick," it is murder, and in a most vicious, cruel and ruthless manner.

After first gasping at the outrageous news that bestial mRNA was approved for insertion into the human genome - that is the "covid vaccine," I was further shocked and appalled when I saw PPE, and the "proning protocol."

At that point I didn't need dancing nurses to convince me that MURDER was the intent behind the Covid "scamdemic."

Proning is so convenient for removing organs, while the patient is **paralysed,** but **not anaesthetised.**

Proning, that is, being forced to lie face down, Is the worst possible position for a patient with respiratory difficulties or in any form of respiratory distress.

The victim is then paralysed by injection.

The victim is *not anaesthetised.*

A vent is inserted in the patient's neck.

The organs are removed rapidly, the patient lying face down, helpless, paralysed, feeling every vicious slice into his or her flesh, the heart being removed last to keep the other organs as fresh as possible.

Finally, highly pressurised oxygen is pushed into the lungs, puncturing them and allowing a death certificate of "respiratory failure" to be issued.

Secret autopsies revealing puncture HOLES in the lungs of "covid" victims were performed in Italy and the USA.

Isn't that special. So "humane."

So "someone else" can live and the medical staff and hospital are $100,000 richer in the space of an hour or two.

This is not a horror movie. If it were, the forecourts of the cinemas would be covered with emesis (vomit) or it would be banned from movie circuits.

The patient is paralysed and so cannot cry out, but witnesses have seen tears flowing from the eyes of those being surgically murdered. I have seen videos, and no, *not* CGI nor AI! The stuff of nightmares, horror movies, demonism...

Intubations guarantee maximum discomfort, least resistance. It is hard to prone intubated patients – forcing them to lay flat and face down, obstructing the movement of the diaphragm, in other words, putting them at high risk of suffocation even before the organs can be sliced out. So vents are inserted via the carotid vein, imposing more suffering and discomfort and further restricting movement.

Remdesivir or Midozalam are prescribed to the patients until the kidneys are destroyed and the lungs become like wet sponges.

At which point oxygen is power-pushed into the lungs, rupturing them.

Secret autopsies in Rome and the USA have found HOLES in the lungs of persons murdered in this manner.

Now there has to be an element of SADISM in murdering patients in such a manner.

80% of surgeons admitted to sadistic fantasies in a 1980's survey – so a profession of sociopaths and psychopaths?

What are the others?

Saints?

Most likely! Or zombies.

It may sound extreme, but any individual who can survive the US Medical training system of sleep deprivation and "on call" service with their humanity intact probably is on his or her way to sanctity!

How can an intelligent mind properly review events, results, "failures," etc., under conditions that are used to control cult members and condition *seasoned, fit,* soldiers or agents to withstand torture.

How can they question protocols, when their funds, their gifts, their text books are written by Pharmashills?

And their professors or Medical Directors own shares?

And are under strict directives.

The Medical Director who applied for a grant to study Homeopathy's effect on respiratory patients was told he could have the grant if he excluded the term "Homeopathy."

If the organ thefts, *not "harvesting," THEFTS,* are not motivated by unmitigated sadism, then the other "chief suspect" is...good old fashioned **greed!**

While there is no "profit" in unsaleable lungs and kidneys, with, and I choke on the words, "lost high market value," there may very well be a personal incentive or satisfaction in abusing patients in such a manner.

Then again, the ghouls can still sell the eyes, brains, livers, etc., of their helpless and hapless victims.

By the refrigerated truckload!

Given the "visuals," i.e. the dearth of dynamic populations in small and large towns, the paucity of children and babies, the windows posting "help wanted" signs for over a year, the closure of small businesses due to lack of staff and lower turnover, i.e., income, the higher number seems closer to the mark.

Thousands and thousands, millions, in fact, were abused and murdered in such a manner.

Persons, citizens, denied the consolation their loved ones' presence, help support. Denied last rites. The slab of beef in the butchers' shops received more respect!

Estimates range from 17 million to 33 million, increasing daily.[11]

And in which "markets" were the eyes, organs, "spare parts" of American citizens sold?

China? Saudi Arabia? Emiratis? Ukraine's dark labs?

But to answer the original question. Yes, it is murder.

And all the excuses for "organ harvesting" (disgusting abuse of terminology!) and transplants, and the rest are completely obliterated by the incredible power of *AUTHENTIC* Homoeopathy!

---

[11] "Mitochondrial Murder has suggestions for the mitigation of some of the most lethal effects of the Covid 19 bioweapon, i.e., anti coagulants such as wine, cinnamon, aspirin, tonic water, etc...

Another reason to hate us.

We do not exploit and profiteer from human suffering.

One more point - aside from Divine miracles, Homeopathy is the singular, only, uniquely *regenerative* protocol, the most thoroughly tested and proven therapeutic system ever!

In other words, we do not harm. Not, first, not second, not final, *not ever! And "Homeopathy works!"*

However, irresponsible prescribing by the amateurs currently courted by Boericke and Tafel's [12] "replacements" discourages those who need us most, as they seldom obtain the best results, and make future Rx a challenge.

And no, we are not "grandma's kitchen remedies" but a gentle, powerful, precise, the most intensively studied and researched protocol of all time; the "hardest medicine to learn and the hardest to practice, *but the most effective!*"

The latter quote is from a statement made directly to me from an MD, who took the time to become a Doctor of Homeopath and Doctor of Oriental Medicine, but "who makes more money as an MD in Vegas." And who can blame him!

The Pharma docs, aka allopaths, get far more respect for handing out dependency meds, suppressive meds, psychotropic meds, than we do for our exquisitely curative and precise Homeopathic potentials.

Like the GP in Ireland who bragged that "(he) can see four or five patients in the time it takes (me) to see one."

At which point I divested him of his delusions and reminded him that mine fully recover while his "stay on the tablets..."

---

[12] The great Homeopathic Pharmacy in Pennsylvania.

And then his secretary started a smear campaign.

I may repeat that story, because it is an interesting metaphor for the controlling ethos of contemporary medicine..." do as we say or *we will destroy you...*

"Befehl ist Befehl" also imported via Operation Paperclip?[iii]

CHAPTER 10 - ORGAN DONATION: Charity – or Grift?

If the Church says that being an organ donor is an "act of charity" with full knowledge of the fact that Fauci brought the *homicidal* proning- paralysing - organ theft - pressurised oxygen pushing techniques from Communist china, then the Church is wrong, wrong, wrong, in deep sin, and must make amends.

Starting with the idolatry of the masks and alcohol gels in the churches and any use of patients as organ donors! The only exception being voluntary partial liver and voluntary kidney transplants, with full and clear explanations to the donor as to the expected outcome and any future proscriptions or limitations on lifestyle.

And then, only after the patient has been offered **authentic** *Homeopathic treatment for the underlying condition.*

Without interference.

It may be just as well that a kidney donor never met the recipient of his so generous gift...

She was grateful, but wished she never accepted it.

Life became so complicated, with anti-rejection drugs, limitations on lifestyle, etc., that the only noticeable effect of the transplant was to severely limit her daily life and function.

A former patient, a nurse working in a dialysis unit, said that the most difficult aspect of her work was sending home patients who seemed in relatively good health and never seeing them again.

In other words, sudden death.

However, hepatic and renal donors are often well intentioned, altruistic persons, acting out of compassion for family members...

However, that compassion can sometimes be manipulated on behalf of strangers – strangers with addictive tendencies, iatrogenic damage, or impairment due to street drug use. On the other hand is it for the benefit of the patient – or of the transplant industry, profiteering from grants, public funds , e.g., Medicaid-Medicare, etc..

It is extremely frustrating to work with a patient ostensibly trying to avoid a transplant but unwilling to give up coffee, opioids, legally prescribed or street, and declining to tell their Homeopath until said Homeopath recognises that the precisely and carefully chosen remedy's action is impaired and impeded.

*In other words, the patient sabotages his or her cure, and, yes, initially lies about dependencies on *harmaceuticals, opioids, coffee, etc.*

Coffee is a mild stimulant, often used to excess, but which, containing small amounts of theophyllin, can be used to open airways in extremis.

However, Coffee, Eucalyptus, Peppermint, Spearmint and other strong odors and flavors can impede and sabotage the effects of our beautiful remedies.

We always advise the patient of these factors, and if the patient expresses concern at being unable to resist the lure of the coffee pot, we can work through the foundations of that and assist the patient to release his or her dependency.

But if he or she does not so advise us, then… it's a frustrating struggle…and an injustice to the Homeopathist as our remedies are cancelled by strong odors or aromas before they can even *begin* to work and we watch with concern as the patient who claims to never take or to have given up coffee, peppermint, etc., shows no signs of symptom change or correction and above all, fails to recover.

This is where *experience* is immensely helpful. Brilliant neophyte may start to doubt their prescriptions, rather than the patient's fidelity to protocols.

"Converts" from "*harma" meds are often the most frustrating to work with.

Medical Director, told to take ONE DOSE of the precisely chosen remedy, calls the following morning with the news that he has consumed the entire "tube" and "what now?" And yes, I did explain our methodology in *detail.*

Kindly nurse sends many gifts, not requested, not required. Meanwhile, no progress with her condition.

Eventually she owns up and admits to being not only a coffee addict but dependent on oxycontin and would prefer to have her bladder removed than give it up.

Experience makes remedy selection a little easier; however, certain remedies have overlapping symptoms so in chronicity it makes all the difference to our patients if we meticulously verify the precise remedy accommodating the **totality of symptoms – in particular the "peculiarities..."**

And thereby save our patients from the agony and indignity of organ removal, replacement and lifelong dependency on anti-rejection drugs.

CHAPTER 11 - HOMEOPATHY FOR CELIBATES

It could be axiomatic to say that by the time they decide to see the "doktah," most patients are depleted and somewhat anxious.

Most patients seem to crave touch.

In a degraded, genitally obsessed world, everything is sexualised - or worse — touch now used as a means of control instead of caress and comfort, as with Meghan Markle's "palm print" crawls up and down Harry's back to "guide" him say, when she wants to leave a place, as an equestrian's knees subtly control their horse during dressage, or like Obama's hand plonked on the biceps of people he wishes to control.

During Covid, Dr. Fauci used the same techniques to control his team, crawling his tiny extremities up and down tall, sturdy, Dr Redfield's back, as if coveting his strength.

Touch, from the time of our birth, becomes intrinsically and extrinsically comforting, re-assuring, even healing, *but must always be appropriate, never controlling nor imposing.*

Homeopaths seldom need to "touch" their patients, but where appropriate, they receive a hug or handshake.[13]

Because touch is healing and comforting, has language of its own and can be diagnostically helpful.[14] That does *not* include inappropriate touching.

Dreading human touch can often indicate a history of trauma, physical or emotional. So that also helps us assist our beloved patients.

---

[13] Where allopathy, e.g., diagnostic xrays, blood tests, etc., fail, the oriental pulses succeed.
[14] "Galvanic skin response," for example.

Our work is analytical. It requires great objectivity on the Homeopath's part, and great subjectivity on the part of our beloved patients.

We require minutiae, symptoms or signs that are scoffed at by the MD or GP, and yet the smallest and least significant symptom can make all the difference between a rapid recovery and a "pedestrian" one.

Persons conditioned to take pills three times a day and accept suppression of symptoms as "cure" have a difficult time accepting that the Homeopath sometimes has to go beyond the apparent symptoms – clearing the acute "pictures' first before delving into chronicity or *causa radica."*

I'm writing "root cause" in Latin because the allopaths are now **copying us – again! Now adopting "root cause" for their own use. Gets tedious!**

Their methodology is one pill for this, another for that... *ad nauseum.*

One Pharmadoc is all over the internet promoting himself as going for "root cause."

Newsflash, buddy, we've been doing that for over two centuries.

With superior results, incomparable statistics and healthier populations.

Where acute conditions are concerned, say, food poisoning, we treat accordingly. However, where there are recurring symptoms, or sensitivities, the "striae" must be removed, uno per uno – the layers peeled back one by one. Requires mutual diligence.

Religious and lay celibates who are vowed to chastity should be most comfortable with our analytical methodologies.

However, I note that many crave touch – not sensual but the comfort of a human to human connection.

There was one Bishop, however, from a distant land, who, seeing me on an overnight to treat a seriously ill patient with trauma based paralysis, let the provincial know that he would like a consult with me.

As soon as I entered the room, he looked me over and said he was having problems with his prostate.

I took out my pen and paper and asked him to recount his symptoms.

He looked extremely disconcerted then said I needed to *"examine"* his prostate. At that point I realised where the "consult" was going, advised him that was not how we worked and left.

That was unusual for a clerical consultation, though as they say in show biz – "there's always one!"

Normally, however, I compensate for our reserved praxis by taking the oriental pulses, *after* taking the case notes.

This is mutually beneficial. It affirms the patient, who sometimes has revealed embarrassing or painful symptoms, and it provides an extra insight into the status of the internal organs and dynamic metabolism.

As I have written elsewhere[15] the most dramatic proof of its efficacy was in determining the origin of pain, i.e., which organ was compromised, when all the "bells and whistles" in NY Hospital's Emergency Room failed!

____

[15] The Tuscany Express – Travels with a Homeopath

The touch there is along both wrists.

CHAPTER 12 - "Syn-Theism" Vs Contra Natura

"Syn-theism" is my word for working *with* the amazing systems gifted by a "Gracious God" to His human children.

Science is the **study of Creation**. Science cannot create a single cell, leaf, drop of rain by thought and intent alone.

Unlike the Creator.

Science only uses all the tools, Gifts, Elements, Systems within the human person and in this great and extraordinary world and planetary system that are already *created* by God!

The "vaccine," the organ theft, the donor racket, abortion, the AZT racket, etc., are NOT the will of God.

How can they be; they are so *contra natura,* so apposite and oppositional to God's benevolent plan for humanity, that they can only be from the dark side.

God did not create zombies. He created cogent, intelligent, loving individuals - though evil too often ambushes and destroys the human heart always attacking His greatest creation, the human soul and its capacity to LOVE.

It is up to HIS creatures, we the people, to choose to do HIS Will and follow HIS Commandments... only ten.

Ten Commandments. Now why are admonitions against idolatry, murder, slander, theft of character, property, spouse, coveting, i.e., jealousy, envy, so hard to understand and follow???

The Will of God is *in* those commandments: "I am the Lord Thy God, thou shalt have no God's before me," yet we deify "soyentists" - whose work is, or more aptly, *should be,* nothing more than the STUDY OF CREATION.

All too often, in this technocratic, idolatry of the bits and bytes age, science in the service of Mammon has become the *parody* of Creation, arrogant, disordered, *homicidal,* ***genocidal*** even.

For example, the simple but awesome method of cooling the earth.

The scientist cannot produce one single cell out of nothing. ***Not one cell!***

The scientist is *not* the Creator, yet increasingly works to *usurp* the work of the Almighty, and, indeed, to destroy it.

From the cloning of a poor sheep, to the vicious experiments involving the theft of cerebral (brain) tissue from babies aborted live, for the purpose of abusing their bodies in the "name of research," Bah, flaming humbug...

How sick is that! And yet Governments and national universities in Canada and Ireland fund and promote this depravity.

Cui bono?

THERE IS NO GOOD OUTCOME.

EVERY EXCUSE FOR THAT DEPRAVED LEVEL OF "research" ***has been covered by the authentic Homeopaths. We've cured those conditions!***

Courageous men and women who sacrifice their own lives and the security of their families to save babies from the sadistic, cruel and horrifying slaughter of abortion are vilified and imprisoned.

The men, "soy-entists" and politicians who engineered the "mitochondrial murder" of 17 million – the lower estimate – to 33 million civilians around the world, walk free. Some are paid $100k to make a one hour lecture...

We idolatrise the masks, we fear this photoshopped "dryer ball" i.e. the covid icon, or image as if it were more powerful than God, the Creator who doesn't even have to blink to get rid of it, if it existed as initially described.

Raise the celestial eyebrow and banish the evils from this world! Soon please!

And "Thou shalt not kill," ie the Fifth Commandment − well... abortion, the death jab/clotshot, the proning-paralysing - high pressure push lung-destroying pressurised oxygen, organ theft, what are they - if not murder? Murder for profit?

Or for a deeper, darker, more sinister purpose.*

And the world goes... hurray for "doctor false cheat."[16]

That is idolatry. Idolatry is *not* the Will of God. It is the radical opposite.

Nothing is more uncomfortable for a patient with respiratory difficulties than being proned, forced to lie face down, the diaphragm compressed, nares, nasal passages obstructed.

As a child with chronic, recurrent, severe respiratory conditions, I could only breathe and sleep sitting upright. Face down would be agony! At the age of eleven I correctly diagnosed the underlying factor for my recurrent pleuro-pneumonias, etc., and was dismissed with patronising amusement by my incompetent GP, who'd puff on his pipe in my room, say, "call if she gets any worse," and then went on to be Dean of Medicine at Trinity College. And then the psyches − "why do you *want* to be sick..." SMH! So "joyful" spending weeks in bed, with only books for company, books read with sore burning eyes, and a mostly resentful mother!

---

[16] My own parody of Fauci's name.

I correctly diagnosed the status of two relatives to another former Dean of Medicine at Trinity, now in Canada.

They died a year later, under orthodox treatment. Where is the logic in poisoning a defenseless, often toxic immune system?

Where is the justification for treating porphyria as bowel cancer and irradiating the sufferer to death, unless, oops, yet another misdiagnosis by yet another TCD Dean of Medicine.

TCD did have a phenomenal Physics and Language department, however. Not a complete loss.

My treatment would not require a year on a morphine drip – no evidence of pain, btw; nor irradiation, for a condition that the Homeopath would treat oh so gently, and effectively.

Requires skill, not the Health Food Store – MD *reductio ad absurdam* of "this for this and that for that..."

So many times, the Inferior School, i.e., the MDs have asked me "what would you give for this condition."

"We treat the patient not the ICD code..."

Totality of symptoms are carefully gathered, minutely assessed, meticulously compared, then followed very carefully.

Disease may be acute, chronic, traumatic. Chronic disease may occur in "layers..." We are happiest when "original symptoms" appear and then we finalise the cure.

"Cure" ist "verboten" in pharma medicine!

My agonising back pain was treated with unlimited high potency pain killers and the admonition "come back if it gets any worse."

It would have been significantly reduced if the 11 year old prodigy was taken seriously.

I was a teenager wondering "how much worse must it get…" To parody the late, great Lewis Carroll[17] "to what degree of "worseness" must this worse and worser become!"

And so, when it came time to enter Med School, I said to myself: "This doesn't work."

Chose Math Physics…

And then I discovered Homeopathy! Back pain gone – still a vulnerability after years of maltreatment, but a viable lifestyle awaited me.

Unlike American MDS, from the ethical era of the *de rigeur* Hippocratic oath, my brother did not return to confer with me about our parents, nor did this paragon of Medicine even advise me that he had begun to treat them, that my father had died, and I do believe that he had called out for me on his death bed, nor did he tell me that my brother was dying – over a three year period.

Both parents succumbed to my brother's treatment within two years.

18 months on radiation for my father and a year on morphine for my mother.

I have no doubt that under my care the outcome would have better, kinder, healthier and the life-span longer, and, again, healthier and more productive.

However, my father, brilliant though he was, was still a "test tube" scientist, and so related better and succumbed to the admonitions of his son, the pharma-doc.

---

[17] Oxford Mathematician and author of Alice in Wonderland, etc.

The Classical, Hahnemannian, Homeopath is light years ahead of that. While the Pharma / "health care" industry has stolen much from the Homeopaths, they cannot begin to address the level of authentic scientific analysis, observational skills and "syntheism" with which we diagnose and treat our patients.

"Syntheism" is my word for working *with* the systems placed in the human person by the Creator, each system working independently, but in complete co-operation and harmony with all created systems. Except under duress.

There were inheritance issues as well, which I did not fight, but, basically, being the genius of an extended family comprising many "pedestrian" MDs, with connections to the *harma industry, via research grants, etc., is a bit like being a lamb surrounded by starving, angry jackals.

An existential threat! Mutual – because if the public knew the beauty, power and authority and authentic science of Homeopathy, the *harmaceutical industry would collapse by, say, 75% - and many hospitals would close – for all the right reasons!

You would not have hundreds of dancing nurses, technicians and MDS ready and willing to throw a sick person on his face, intubate and cut out his or her organs. The truth will out!

Nor would you have the "dark humor" common to these practitioners. Alien to Homeopathy!

Sadly there will always be a desire for "heroic medicine" as Homeopaths refer to the Pharma system which requires considerable "heroism," stoicism, submission, on the part of its patients, and the 25% residual pharmacopeia can be useful in extreme accidents and desperate procedures.

There is a lesson there to, for parents "playing favorites." Entitlement leads to arrogance thence to indifference, thence to callousness, the callous indifference that cost them their lives.

The "discarded" children can make a choice: focus on anger, and its sidekick, vengeance, the dish best served cold," or focus on compassion.

If the Church says that being an organ donor is an "act of charity" with full knowledge of the fact that Fauci brought the proning- paralysing - organ theft - pressurised oxygen pushing lung rupturing techniques from Communist china, then the church is wrong, wrong, wrong, in deep sin, and must make amends. Starting with the idolatry of the masks and alcohol gels!

The methods used for "treating" "Covid" are the methods used for removing organs from living political prisoners in China.

Was "covid19" an extrinsic virus, or "vaccinosis" from the mass "vaccinations" aggressively promoted at the onset of the high travel seasons – Thanksgiving, Christmas, etc.?

If those spokespersons for the Church are ignorant of those methods used, then they are at fault for not keeping up with the techniques used in these vile institutions by these ghoulish surgeons, licensed and determined to kill.

(Yes, credit to good surgeons and caring hospitals where credit is due, and while these are not targets of my concern, they appear to be very rare creatures indeed! Sad to say, too many of the better physicians, the "Hippocratic Oath" generation of Physicians who put their patients first, and did not push the mRNA bioweapon and who were personally known to me, have retired or been coerced into retirement.)

CHAPTER 13 – Covid and Criminal Transplant

The speed at which NY Hospitals ran out of paralysands cries out for Federal Investigation.

Likewise, the skewed logistics regarding "co-morbidities" and extreme mortality rate among the elderly.

Yes, I am asking for a serious and intense inquiry into the likelihood that Senior Citizens were murdered in NY Hospitals, *subsequent* to the removal of their organs. Perhaps, under the transplanted, wannabe transgender, Dr Richard aka Rachel Levine, this may have occurred in PA.

I also demand to know why patients with conditions considered so extreme as to "require" transplants are not given the option of *authentic* Homeopathic treatment in order to avoid it.

Paralysing agents, probably including curare derivatives, are used in the removal of organs from living patients, a common practice in China, and reportedly in the USA.

However, anaesthesia is verboten.

Silent tears fall from the victims' eyes as they are systematically butchered for their organs by men and women in white coats, pretending to the world that they are serving suffering humanity while actually salivating over the new car, or house, or vacation "earned" by this crime crying out to Heaven for Justice.

Or do they just revel in the power of usurping the Divine Will, the sole authority over life and death.

Did Fauci bring this criminal practice from China to the USA?

PA's Sec of Health is a man who pretends he is a woman. Whether he believes it or just wants the world to believe is another matter, but it speaks to the mental health and motivation of Richard aka Rachel Levine. Or is he a fugitive from justice?

Added to that, his experience is primarily with minors with alleged eating disorders in New York City. I have considerable experience with the corruption and evil of NYC and NYS' corruption and venality toward the dying and the abuse of anorectics in the 1980s.

Richard, aka Rachel Levine, the doctor who does not know the difference between male and female, but who controlled PA's Health Services during the scamdemic, needs to be held accountable. For manslaughter, if not outright murder! In compromising the health and lives of PA's Senior Citizens, Levine's actions are questionably consistent with those of the dying State of NY, a State executed by its own Governor. -30-

(February 2021)

Addendum: The "Spanish" flu of 1917-1918 was started by the first mass vaccination in the world. It caused 675,000 deaths in the USA – a very loose and conservative estimate.[18]

"Covid," likewise. But the estimated fatalities worldwide were between 17,000,000 and 33,000,000 the latter number being the most plausible.

The shutdown of workers across the USA and the worst hit European nations; the faked death certificates, the abortifacient properties of the mRNA "vaccine" and the refusal by the authorities to do autopsies and admit the horrendous number of death by vascular blocking adhesions, or adhered fibrins pushed into circulation and thence into the heart lead to one dark and dire conclusion:

---

[18] https://www.healthaffairs.org/content/forefront/measuring-mortality-pandemics-1918-19-and-2020-21

"Covid" was an instrument in the depopulation and genocide of the intelligent, productive, white Euro Christian peoples!

Along with abortion, contraception, abortive contraceptives such as IUD and the desperate, cruel and sadistic murders of IVF babies!

After all, $100k per raided, violated corpse and sale of organs extracted from a helpless, chemically paralysed human person, can put a deposit on a fancy home, buy two super cars, an editor, publisher, politician, etc.

But will the "Fed Ex" driver ever recover from the sight of a box of baby eyes breaking open and...

CHAPTER 14 - Covid19 – Lies, Damn Lies and Statistics!

Once upon a time, well after there "were wolves in Wales," and long after the "birds in red flannel petticoats" had flown the pond and become "cardinals" in the Colonies, there were "Cowboys and Indians." Political correctness then gave us "good sheriffs" and "Bad Barts."

Right and wrong became personal constructs. There were no longer any absolutes, just subjective "feelings," "relationships" and "identities." Identity politics replaced any concept of morality.

If it "felt good," it was good!

Because Bolsheviks flooded into the USA, disguised as poor, pathetic refugees, and took over the educational system, and the hearts and minds of our children and terrorized the authentic refugees from Soviet Communism, systematically working their way up from Kindergarten aides to Deans of Ivy League Universities.

Suddenly "one plus one" no longer equaled two, but was replaced by a convoluted narrative - a long series of words in place of numbers and confusing our children.

The parents, accustomed to common sense Math, were baffled and clueless and could not help the children with "Common Core" aka gobbley de gook pseudo Math.

This, along with contemptuous TV "comedies" denigrating adults and aimed at children contributed to a lack of respect and trust in parents and a *reliance* on external parties, i.e., Marxist teachers, to guide the minors to success in their exams and other endeavours.

Numerical computations became an exasperating narrative of anomalous, polysyllabic word strings, aka "word salads!"

Deborah Birx is an outstanding example of its mind numbing psy ops as she clenches her fists, Pelosi-Clinton style, and reiterates misappropriated polysyllables such as "granulation" for her charts and diagrams which showed nothing of disease progression or human suffering. Certainly no sign of relief!

For me, she is forever associated with the term: "Lies, damned lies and statistics," that is, statistics useless for the care and treatment of the suffering, but essential for the *tracking* of the "failed" that is, homicidal CV19 vaccine, to ensure that CV 2020 blooms just in time for maximum damage on Nov 3, 2020.[19]

Math is its own language: unique, direct and highly informative. It does not need awkward and portentious patois. But we know that. Speaking multiple "Romance" languages simultaneously or in rapid sequence might be fun for a while, but is not recommended as a method of instruction and results in gibberish.

"Gibberish" is derived from "gibbet" or apparatus from which humans were once hanged. A "flibberdigibbet" was an evil spirit who flew by the gibbets seeking to capture the dying soul and take him to hell. Gibberish may well be the language of the terrified, or the language of the dark side.

Where Birx,' Fauxci's, Redfield's and Hahn's "sound and fury signifying nothing" gibberish is concerned, the "dark side" seems to be the most likely source.

Unlike the UK where creativity and independent thought was encouraged, the NY Public School teachers found a way to make discovery and education an onerous, punitive, exercise in conditioning children to fill out forms and "just follow orders." This transformation was instigated by the Bolsheviks who infiltrated the USA disguised as "refugees." Does this sound

---

[19] Election set up to deny Trump a 2nd term.

familiar? Oh yes, there were authentic refugees...but allegedly the Obama sponsoring Pritzkers[20] were not in the patriot brigade.

Bad Bart suddenly became the "good guy," the victim, and the "Good Sheriff" was now the villain...how *dare* he love his country, his constitution, history, traditions, family and law and order! And shock, horror, dismay, the Good Sheriff carried a *gun!* Bad Bart's guns were ignored along with every incendiary item including words and ideology!

And so, the "Good Sheriff" comes into town, takes out the bad guys, makes the streets safe for work, for leisure, for enterprise and brings it all back to life,

And when the people start to cheer,

In comes Bad Bart, with a mask and a sneer.

The weak cower in fear – and blame the Good Sheriff.

And so, to show Bad Bart they're on his side, they wear a mask and jeer.

And plant their roadblocks everywhere.

The manner in which vents were used may have caused more fatalities than the CV "virus," aka "vaccinosis." Proning patients, sedating or paralyzing them puts them at risk of clots, and pushing pressurized oxygen into damaged lungs is sadistic insanity – unless the intent is death, in which case it is homicidal, criminal in fact! [iv]

Proning is agonising for patients with respiratory conditions, but is also the preferred method for stealing organs. Don't call it "harvesting."

---

[20] Pritzkers were allegedly Bolshevik agents who entered the USA as "refugees" from the USSR.

We "harvest" that which we have planted and nurtured until it is ripened.

That is not what happens with "organ theft!"

The donor is murdered during the act of retrieval!

Accident and trauma victims are most valuable – often young and fit with healthy organs.

Healthy organs and shocked, traumatised family members are also easy marks when it comes to signing away their loved one's organs, trying to bring some benefit from the pain, suffering and bereavement, but instead, unknowingly subjecting their loved ones to unspeakable agony, repeat *unspeakable.*

Like the slaughtered pre-natal babies whose vocal cords are sliced by the abortionists, they cannot cry out, nor express their anguish.

Why upset the doktahs, the nurses, the ghouls, the "transplant"team"" with the effect of their sadistic and cruel practices.

Sadistic, cruel and **unnecessary practices.**

IN 2024 my concerns are now justified. "Covid" hysteria and the subsequent mass murder of toxified humanity, iatrogenically hybridised by bestial mRNA subsequent to systematic destruction of kidneys by iatrogenic medicines such as Remdesivir, killed between 17 and 33 million human persons, from pre-natal babies to geriatric patients, isolated and separated from their loved ones, dying alone and uncherished.

"First Do No Harm!" is the first admonition of the Hippocratic Oath.

But my Church was silent!

CHAPTER 15 - Infertility

Major causes of infertility include: natural or inherited pathologies, environmental disease, malnutrition, obesity, poor physical health, harmful or inadequate living conditions, prolonged use of oral contraceptives, IUDs, [21] previous abortions, violence or abuse and, sometimes, psychological trauma and grief.

Homeopathy can address and promote the recovery and repair of the reproductive system, gently and without ignominious and physically intrusive examinations, as well as helping women who suffered from spontaneous miscarriages to carry their babies to term.

Sometimes our questions might appear "impertinent" or not relevant to the particular area of concern, but every symptom contributes to the precise prescription required for the most rapid recovery.

Again, acute cases usually respond to Homeopathy with amazing "agility." Chronic cases need more time, although positive changes are usually quickly apparent.

Treat the dominant systems first.

If relative to emotional trauma, treat those first. The entire process of abortion is demeaning, destructive, dangerous and a repeat of the rape process.

The mother is made to strip, put her feet in stirrups while the abortionist probes her reproductive organs, inserts plugs, knives, "vaccuum cleaner" extensions or whatever s/he considers the fastest and most effective way of murdering the

---

[21] Inter uterine devices, implanted in utero, often for years, removed with tissues of dead embryos clinging thereon. IUD are de facto abortifacients!

little baby, according to time of gestation, while his-her assistant watches.

This is usually another female, who then inserts drips, anaesthetics, and turns on the powerful suction machine, which tears the infant to pieces, and suctions out the little embryonic baby in pieces, along with the blood supply and possibly part of the uterine lining.

This causes shock, physical harm, cardiac arrest, emotional trauma.

The brutal forcing of the "green," or unripe cervix can cause the loss of future children.

Many women experience dissociation, that is, they suppress the memory of the abortion until the sound of a vacuum cleaner suddenly triggers the sufferer.

Perhaps on the anniversary of the due date, or of the abortion.

Because dissociation is a powerful coping method for unbearable suffering, guilt or regret.

Another term or variation is "Stockholm Syndrome."

The six year young niece and child bride of Mohammed lived in that "walled in state" until she reached the age of 19 and Mohammed brought another six year old into the house for the same abusive treatment and she "snapped."

Interestingly, overwhelmed by rage, pain, fear at what was done to her, and to protect the other child, she proceeded to poison Mohammed. In other words, he was killed by the niece that he molested for three years from the age of six and raped when the molestations triggered premature menarche.[22]

---

[22] Menarche – onset of first menses

Something his adherents refuse to admit.

There is no record of Mohamhead having children with Ayesha, but the possibility of traumatic damage to internal organs is high, making the poor child infertile.

Dickens was a great proponent of Homeopathy and his female characters provide intriguing "symptom pictures" concommitant with our remedies.

I will put their remedies in random order at the back for those who are interested...[v]

<u>Great Expectations.</u>

Miss Havisham – stuck in the past, cold, even ruthless.... mice still nibbling on a twenty year old wedding cake...(movie version) Periods stopped due to the shock of betrayal.

Estella – beautiful, but cold and calculating... that picture is incomplete...and falls between three remedies...depending on cause and other concommitants...

Mrs. Gargery – resentful, complaining, bitter even...angry but not ruthless...

<u>Pickwick Papers:</u>

Mrs. Pocket – Obliging, charming, loving, children "tumbling out of her pockets..."

Mrs. Pocket appears to be the same affectionate prototype as **Peggotty** in David Copperfield.

<u>David Copperfield</u>

Peggotty, a servant, loves children, puts her own status at risk in order to comfort young David before he is packed off to boarding school.

Peggotty and Mrs. Pocket are unlikely to have fertility issues, but may be susceptible to frequent miscarriage.

Another remedy which I associate with Queen Victoria also has the rubric – "easy conception, easy loss..."

After a few losses and genetically impaired babies due to marriage with her first cousin, Albert, Queen Victoria consulted Homeopaths.

The courage of desperation - as Homeopathy was still very new, but in gratitude for the success of Homeopathy, she gave us a Royal Charter, facilitated the opening of Homeopathic Hospitals and potentially saved millions of lives.

So if we get to Heaven and see her there, it will be for that reason, and not for the gluttony and indifference to the death by starvation of millions of Irish in the mid and late 19th century under the Norman lords and the suffering and untimely deaths of English children on London's streets and in the great displacements by the "dark, satanic mills..."

Again – gluttony...sin or syndrome?

Symptom of mineral deficiency, mal absorption, digestive disorder.

Mal absorption often points to a fundamental cause of infertility and / or difficulty in carrying a sweet baby to term.

Mal absorption of calcium or iron compounds, or deficiency, in, say, intrinsic factor, zinc, etc,can also lead to severe anemia, thence, difficulty in conception, infertility, birth anomalies or frequent miscarriage.

It is risky to list the names of the Homeopathic potentials, as Big *harma tends to grab, control, misuse, abuse, etc., in order to discredit our incredible arsenal of deeply researched remedies derived from the canopy of the earth, so intricately interacting, co-existent with humanity for centuries, sharing the same contingencies, catastrophes, *Divinely endowed cellular intelligence...*

As I hopefully conclude this book on the Feast Day of St. Francis of Assisi, I note that the most humble of plants is often the most powerful at eliminating the most complex of cellular errors, the exotic orchid having the most limited applications in our Repertory, while the most humble and accessible of plants obtain the most outstanding results in the darkest of diseases.

CHAPTER 16 – Human Life International

Copy of message sent to HLI on May 29 2024

Whose side are you on?

(You)did not publish my Comment made on May 28, 2024. I am probably the singular Homeopath left on this planet with the skill and in-hospital experience, *qua* Homeopath, in:

- restoring sensation, movement, life to paralysed limbs;
- weaning patients off respirators,
- permanently stopping recurrent seizures in a child three thousand miles away,
- rapidly restoring speech to non-verbal children.
- Rapidly healing MRSA
- Rapidly clearing Hep A,B,C, viral load 100% in patients around the world.
- Bringing patient out of coma – (not on official record)
- Accelerating symphysis in fractures, inc. an octogenerian with osteoporosis.

I warned about the extreme dangers of the Neuralink. I'm already blocked from Twitter/X.

I "wonder why."

How in God's name was that evil "thing" allowed to progress.

So, as my high level English friends say "when are you coming home?" and "why hasn't the world heard from you yet?"

You might ask the same, re my rather "shocking" achievements.

"Shocking" because in a sane world I would be given the support and encouragement to help so many suffering persons, but instead, I've been "hunted" by corrupt and venal magistrates in Montgomery County, largely owned by Pfizer-GSK, and a fake substitute "judgette" in WA, although that had more to do with a property grab on the part of the new Saudi owners, implanting their jihadis across the pleasant towns of the USA and Europe, and evicting all Christians, Seniors, Military than with my practice and hostile *Harma, as far as I know.

And yes I have received calls from well-spoken moslem women, arrogant, entitled, insistent, obviously educated in the West, seeking advice for "treatments" of wounds in the desert.

Notably *snake bites.*

One in particular was very insistent, and like a Columbia U communist Professor, found my unlisted home phone number by some devious means. She could not or would not understand the highly specific and precise methodologies that we use to treat our patients and tried to use our potentials while bypassing our protocols. I resisted the temptation to allow that, especially with the snake venoms in our "arsenal." I refuse to betray Homeopathy.

There are several types of snake venom, most are haemorrhagic, but some are thrombotic. 36 found in positive "covid" tests!

The Lord, in His Mercy, made snakes that cause bleeding, and those that cause clotting.

Bleeding in a limited manner allows the body to expel any explicit or covert venoms contained from the snake's poison sacs.

Clotting then stops the bleeding.

That's somewhat simplistically expressed.

If not managed, clots or thromboses can create other problems, particularly if induced by allopathic medicines.

We do not kill our snakes, just milk the venom, and triturate and dynamise it. "Less is more" applies doubly where the "herpetic" symptoms occur.

Snake venoms must never be taken for granted nor used casually, even in the Homeopathic dilutions.

A "Society" MD fraudulently practicing Homeopathy prescribes *fifteen high potency remedies per day to a patient, including the microdiluted venoms.*

Her patient, a beautiful young woman, had a diagnosis of cancer of the uterus, and while Homeopaths have treated "cancer" with great success, when the system is not too compromised by the chemo-radiation, an authentic Homeopath would never prescribe in such a manner!

All this has led to people saying "I tried Homeopathy but / and it didn't work."

A few questions reveal the fact that while a Homeopathic remedy-potential was used, it was used improperly, more or less as an allopathic Rx, eg., TID, three times a day!

Only in acute cases, matey! And say, in food poisoning from decaying matter, two doses of the correct remedy will usually suffice.

In other words they did not "try" Homeopathy at all.

Homeopathy misused by an allopath is neither Homeopathy nor allopathy, just plain FRAUD.

This woman was a sweet and kind young person, who loved children. However, deceived by the "anything goes" post Woodstock generation into accepting a secondary lifestyle, that is mistress to a succession of high level executives, and the consequent insistence on termination, by the time she reached her mid-thirties she had multiple abortions.

In spontaneous abortion, that is, natural interruption of pregnancy, the reproductive systems and "recovery" systems are prepped and primed for the loss of the baby.

The cervix opens naturally; it is not forced open. The cells stop multiplying.

Note the chimerical fetal cells stay within the mommy after birth...but they are still within the mother pre-birth, "informing" her body of the needs and requirements of the wee baby.

Just as, post birth, the nipple is sensitised to the saliva of the baby and triggers a response for the provision of any lacks, wants or needs, perceived from the saliva.

Probably why the Creator put such a concentration of sensors in the lingual, sublingual, parotid, mandibular, facial, trigeminal nerves aka the "straps."

And, it would appear, "transmitters" as well!

The level of transcellular communication and extra conscious perception in the central nervous systems of the human body is phenomenal.

Back to the effects of traumatically removing a wee baby from his or her mother before his or her time...

The baby's trauma is well documented. At least by pro-Lifers and those actively engaged in the homicide of pre-natal infants.

*"It is hard to convince yourself that you are not taking a human life when you are **throwing little arms and legs into a bucket...**"*

"Doktahs" are expected to be intelligent, so how many decades and how many IQ points were required before "Dr." Bernard

Nathanson recognised that tearing the arms and legs of a wee baby in his or her Divinely ordained "safe place" was not only **murder, but murder of the most vicious and sadistic nature.**

So vicious, so sadistic, that its true nature has been kept from the media and general public!

SC Justices, professors, journalists and even "deathscorts" have no idea that the "Right" they sustain, propose or legalise, is criminal, sinful, barbaric, sa*anic - unadulterated and vicious evil.

Even the Barbarians believed that killing babies was a way of propitiating the "gods," *de facto demons,* and was directed for the "benefit" of the tribe.

Note how child sacrificing tribes die, hoist on their own bloody petards.

Today, abortions are a matter of "convenience" and "public image..."

The majority of first time abortions are done under duress. Ironically duress by the future grandmothers... in laws or blood mothers of the "accidentally pregnant" mother.

I know for a fact that some of those mothers were in cults and were sacrificed in childhood...to paedophiles, etc., in sick and bizarre rituals.

They were all terrified of their birth mothers.

Some had multiple abortions by the time they reached their twenties.

All wanted to keep their babies but were too terrified to resist for long.

I watched one sobbing in my consulting rooms in NY, such a sweet girl...the more options I offered to her, the deeper and louder the sobs.

She was 24, raised in a cult, would never get away from the mother who controlled her — so liberal that said mother was "expelled" from the Social Work Program at a NY University in the first semester of her Freshman year.

So sad that her adult daughter could not also "expel" her!

SO MUCH FOR CHOICE AND SELF DETERMINATION!

CHAPTER 17 – Post Abortion Syndrome

In mid and late term abortions, the mother feels the baby kick and back away from the MD Butcher's knife.

By "trauma" I include *the travesty of induction, of violence, either surgical or blunt trauma, or by poisonous chemicals, pharmaceutical toxins, "accredited" by the very agencies installed to protect us from such abominations.*

So baby is removed, but the mother's body is "geared" to carry that baby for 9.5 -10 months during which the Human chorionic Gonadatrophin levels can remain high, and as they support cell replication can lead to abnormal growths in the uterus[23] and potential future molar pregnancies[24].

There are many sources other than those designated in the footnotes but while they continue to refer to a baby as the "fetus" they will deliberately or unconsciously refuse to see or acknowledge the devastating effects of abortion on the female reproductive system, and the mind, heart – and for Christians, *soul* – of persons involved in or acquiescing to, the deliberate, pre-meditated slaughter of the human prenatal baby.

And what an insult to the exquisite and Divine design of the physiology of women...and men, and the symbioses essential and intrinsic to the survival of the Human Race.

Abortion kills a baby's body. It shatters a woman's soul. I try not to judge, especially when not in consultation, but once recognised, Post Abortion Syndrome is hard to deny.

---

[23] https://my.clevelandclinic.org/health/articles/22489-human-chorionic-gonadotropin
[24] https://my.clevelandclinic.org/health/diseases/17889-molar-pregnancy

PAS women are nine times as likely to attempt suicide as the general population.

PAS women can go for years, in denial, in dissociation, until, suddenly the sound of a vacuum aspirator (sterilised vacuum cleaner, basically,) brings her to tears. Or, more precisely, brings the hidden tears to the surface, with heart rending sobs.

I see it in the eyes of men at Pro Life rallies, the shock, anger, bewilderment of men who begged for and promised the world to the mother of their child if she would save their baby...and found they had NO RIGHTS whatsoever over their progeny.

Could look at it this way.

The mother works for 9.5 months to gestate her baby.

The father works for the rest of his life to care for mother and child.

That's the way our Creator planned it and the way His Nature orders it...

But suddenly the Western Middle classes were becoming educated, prosperous and a challenge to elitist power bases. Legalised abortion doubled the workforce and halved the wages!

And the feminist movement convinced women that it was their "Right" and obligation to become inferior versions of men, leaving the comforts of home and family to enter dangerous and disquieting occupations, leaving their children to fend for themselves.

"Rights" for women completely voided the Rights and protections for children, Rights and protections validated throughout centuries.

Rights for mothers, Rights for Fathers, Right to Kill and Destroy the "product" of their love for one another.

Until the vile, decadent, syphilitic[25] retchingly filthy communists upended it.

Using the word: "RIGHTS." Turning the amazing Constitution of the USA on its head!

Women experiencing more than one abortion are most likely to abuse their children. And / or abandon them.

Every year a Post Abortion mother experiences two devastating anniversaries.

These would be the "due date" or birthdate of the murdered child, and the death date, or date of abortion termination of the murdered infant.

Play all the word games you like: zygote, blastocyte, embryo, fetus, a *baby is a baby no matter how small!*

23 Chromosomes from Mom, 23 from Dad. A unique and irreplaceable human person!

One of a kind. Never to appear on this earth again.

Each with a unique Gift and challenge from the Creator.

Sometimes the "Gift" is the challenge, and the "challenge," the Gift!

The builder constructs a wall.

---

[25] Every leading Communist, Socialist, psycho Sadistic Monarch or dictator suffered from tertiary syphilis. Hitler, Stalin, Marx, Mao, etc. And filthy habits. Henry VIII infected his wives and children, lost a few babies as a result. Elizabeth II covered her face with thick, lead paste, was sterile, probably not "Virgin."

He orders a certain number of bricks, each uniquely numbered for a specific location in the wall.

A jealous "competitor" hijacks the delivery truck and smashes the bricks.

The workers continue to build the wall, but without the assigned bricks it keeps tumbling down.

A baby is a baby no matter how small!

Even "Dr Seuss" knows that!

And he's a cat!!

A cat in a hat! Just fancy that!!!

He isn't a doctor - not a doctor at all,

*But he knows that <u>a baby's a baby **no matter how small!**</u>*

I'd trust Dr. Seuss over Planned Parenthood's butchers! Any day!

And the MDs who promote and endorse abortion are now demoted far below the level of a fictitious, cartoon cat, because they do not know a "baby is a baby" until, like their leading businessman – MD, Bernard Nathanson, they ask "why are we throwing little arms and legs into a bucket?" If we are not taking human life?

When we murder peacemakers, spiritual leaders, priests, bishops, teachers, AUTHENTIC scientists, community leaders, artists, musicians, in utero, our communities, nations, towns, cities, parishes, must be rebuilt, time and time again.

Until we *get the message!*

Or Armageddon ensues!

It is God's world, God's wall, and He has a plan for each and every one of us that he sends into this world, a plan that is exquisite in its minutiae...

So exquisite, that the structure, the interpretation is exclusive only to our Saints, the most spiritually advanced and enlightened persons in the Universe...

Saints, having the challenging honor of living with their minds in Celestia and their feet on the humble, fertile, generous, life giving despised earth, live the Unitive way, in complete harmony with the will and desire of the Lord.

They have learned the language which the "Illuminatives" and "Purgatives" struggle with, and guide those of us less Gifted in spiritual matters, in the Way of the Lord.

But how many were murdered in utero?

What have we done!

We've ruptured the foundations of our earthly home, built walls without bricks, castles without foundations, cathedrals without 'bells," etc...

CHAPTER 18 – "No Good Deed..."

"No good deed goes unpunished!"

That stands true for all the pro- Lifers harassed or imprisoned for defending and protecting helpless pre-natal infants by such "infamous" methods as standing and praying outside baby butchering abattoirs, handing leaflets guiding to safe places and support for mothers, and persevering in the dissemination of the truth and facts about abortion.

No Presidential medals of honor in the USA for my phenomenal work in Goldwater Memorial Hospital, just an ambush on the streets of New York, August 16, 2006, and Nov 2, 2006. NYPD saved my life but were not allowed to investigate - and "fuggadabout" the corrupt NY prosecutors, and judiciary. Most likely enjoying dividends from investment in PP and Big *harma.

As I said back in the 1970s - the first generation to promote abortion would be the first to be forcibly "euthanised." More like "dysthanised" if you look clearly at the death toll from the genocidal bestial-human mRNA "vaccines" and the suffocating effects of the "euthanasia" pills.

At the first mention of mRNA I knew that it would be easier to antidote Zyclon B than this deadly putrefaction.

I expected some leadership from the Vatican.

But the Church was silent - except for our rare and wonderful saints on the ground...

Which leads me to deeply question the motivation for said silence.

And the degree to which Archdioceses and so called "Catholic" charities may be invested in Big *harma.

But I have to wonder at HLI. Their book on Cosmetics and Fetal Cells also claimed that "vaccines made from (butchered baby) cell lines" can be permitted by the RC Church because they "save lives."

Sorry, but you are WRONG, WRONG, WRONG.

There is no justification for abortion, "fetal cell lines," "fetal cell testing," etc. Those are fake justifications for the murder of human infants and the other ghoulish research for which these sweet babies are sacrificed.

Every "flu epidemic" FOLLOWS the "flu vax season." Oh Mia Mama Maria! How wrong do you have to be, HLI? Svegliarte!

Or will you wait until "Neuralink"chips are enforced on healthy citizens, or start dislodging into the circulation and the cardiac valves... will the diagnosis be "rupture" or will they stick with the worn "myocarditis" diagnosis?

And *why in Heaven's name do Catholic Hospitals ignore the "Gift of a Gracious God?"*[26]

Cardinal O'Connor tried, set up a meeting with his Health care managers, but we were sabotaged by a manufacturer of Homeopathic remedies...who must have done a "deal with the devils" in the NIH and FDA.

Said Health Care managers were no blessing either, two large women, obviously friendly with Big *harma.

Boiron was handed a gift on a silver platter but Thierry Boiron, educated in an American college, put down every suggestion, in a way that I can only describe as ... *French!* Gestures, shrugs...

Ironically, the allopath, the Medical Director of a major NY Hospital and myself were exchanging glances of shocked

---

[26] Hahnemann's description of Homeopathy

incomprehension...as the heir to one of the largest and most famous Homeopath "Pharmacies" was sabotaging the biggest opportunity that we had in decades – the best part of a century, in fact!

CHAPTER 19 - Idolatry and Covid

Was the Church guilty of idolatry in the time of Covid?

The EU "exemptions" for the mRNA "vaccine" included Medical Professionals, Media, Diplomats, Executives...

It is just "coincidental" that the EU President, Ursula von Leyen, is the daughter or granddaughter of one of Hitler's Senior SS officers, i.e., a wee "Gestapo Girl."

Her predecessor, Angela Merkel, is Hitler's daughter, and formerly employed by East Germany's Stasi, or secret police. Fourth Reich? And allegedly Obama's aunt. Photos do lie nowadays, but the photo of Merkel smiling benevolently on her young "nephew," Obama appeared 100% genuine.

Seeing a pattern here? Von Leyen's husband is Pfizer's EU VP in charge of "vaccine" distribution.

And then there is "Operation Paperclip." And the world was silent, as America's then President, Harry Truman, brought the vilest ghouls in the history of science, to continue their lethal research projects in the Land of the Free and the Home of the Brave.

While the bereaved and exhausted Americans celebrated the end of the war or continued to rebuild their lives with breaking hearts and "gold stars[27]" on their houses, 1,600 Nazi scientists landed in the USA, were welcomed by officials, and given every facility, means and money to continue the evil research started under Adolph Hitler aka Herr Schickelgruber in the country that he debased and abused; the land of Bach, Beethoven, Schiller, Schubert, Muller, Goethe - and must we mention Wagner - .that the "little Austrian" turned into a murder machine!

---

[27] A gold star on the wall of a house represents a fallen military hero.

Back to "idolatry."

I am Catholic.

As a Catholic I believe that Christ is present in the Eucharist and that all life is beholden, through Him to the Creator.

We know from the scriptures and the hundreds of thousands of miracles occurring daily since the Birth of Christ, or Nativity, that when a case is beyond even Homeopathy's amazing *curative* capacity, that Christ may "Say just the word" and the suffering, the wound, physical or emotional or spiritual, or the infection or trauma, or poison, will dissipate and the patient shall be healed.

So why were our prelates walking up the church aisles, masked to the nines, spewing pathogens, replacing blessed water with dehydrating gels, and basically making a statement, to wit to who, that "Christ has no power."

Oh they of little Faith!

Or, "they" of compromise with Federal monies pouring into "Catholic" hospitals? In exchange for "compliance" with Federal Rules!!!

Or they of "we just luuuurve our Pfizer – GSK – ModeRNA – J and J – Astra Zeneca DIVIDENDS!

If only every God fearing Christian would just dump their stock in the foregoing...

And if only the Federal Government in the USA and their equivalents in other nations would **stop funding highly profitable but destructive private enterprise!**

We just might have a more ethical, honorable world!

And fewer chronically ill people dependent on suppressive and destructive medications.

Which create side effects requiring increasing doses and selections of more suppressive and destructive medications. Until the patient ends up in the ER, or the OR, having a hip "replaced" or a patella (knee) removed, leading to dependence on suppressive and destructive medications for the rest of their lives!

Which is why, sometime in the 1980s the word "cure" was banished from the pharmaco-medical dialogue, and replaced by "maintenance" medicine and "palliative care."

CHAPTER 20 – Silencing of the Shepherds - *Slaughter of the Lambs...*

OUR CHURCH WAS SILENT – why?
Our Pope wore a mask
Our bishops were masked
Our priests were masked
They held up the Sacred Host with sterilised hands – insulting the Healer – Indivisible Son of the Creator, to Whom *all powers were given...*

In the meantime: The EU exempted all Media, Diplomats, Health Care executives, Corporate Executives, etc. from "mandatory mask wearing" and mandatory vaccinations.

How many civilians, salt of the earth doing the "menial" jobs without which the world would plunge into chaos, how many millions were killed by the mRNA bioweapon and are still at risk of loss of life as the accursed fibrins break off – or, worse - replicate?

How many babies were murdered? Senior citizens? Mentally ill and disabled – sound familiar, all ye historians of 1939 onward?

How many who were misdiagnosed, intentionally, because we are now more valued for our organs than for our minds.

And where was the Free Will, the Freedom of Conscience? Any Freedom? We were all under house arrest - not free at all!

Young people, children, teenagers were locked down under house arrest, during years critical to social development, while small businesses folded, land was surreptitiously snatched by foreign "investors." Invaders flooded across the border and parents lost their jobs and self- sufficiency, leading to loss of self-esteem, family tensions and dependence on social services.

Meanwhile, in DC and Pennsylvania:
- Biden administration not mandating COVID vaccines for White House staff, Psaki says
- https://www.breitbart.com/politics/2021/08/12/report-confidential-documents-reveal-pfizer-does-not-mandate-vaccines-for-employees/
  https://thehill.com/changing-america/well-being/prevention-cures/550394-nih-chief-says-he-is-not-requiring-his-employees
- https://sagaciousnewsnetwork.net/the-cdc-does-not-require-its-employees-to-be-vaccinated/
- modeRNA did not mandate it up until the FDA "approved it" so they reversed their policy
- https://www.bizjournals.com/boston/news/2021/08/20/moderna-covid-19-vaccine-staff-mandate.html
  permalink parent / save report block reply

TrudopesEyebrow [S] 2 points 2 hours ago +2 / -0

- https://africacheck.org/fact-checks/fbchecks/yes-astrazenecas-covid-19-vaccine-made-genetically-modified-chimpanzee-virus
- CDC admits the vaccine contains 'aborted human fetus cells'

- https://www.health.nd.gov/sites/www/files/documents/COVID%20Vaccine%20Page/COVID-19_Vaccine_Fetal_Cell_Handout.pdf

permalink parent /save report block reply

PART TWO

CHAPTER 21 – Why Homeopathy?

Courageous men and women who sacrifice their own lives and the security of their families to save babies from the sadistic, cruel and horrifying slaughter of abortion are vilified and imprisoned.

The men, "soy-entists" and politicians who engineered the "mitochondrial murder" of 17 million – the lower estimate – to 33 million civilians around the world, walk free. Some, like Fauci, are reportedly paid $100k to make a one hour lecture...

We idolatrise the masks, we fear this photoshopped "dryer ball" i.e. the covid icon, or image as if it were more powerful than God, the Creator who doesn't even have to blink to get rid of it, if it existed as initially described.

Raise the celestial eyebrow and banish the evils from this world! Soon please!

And "Thou shalt not kill," ie the Fifth Commandment. Well...abortion, the death jab/clotshot, the proning-paralysing-high pressure push lung-destroying pressurised oxygen... what is that, if not murder?

Murder for profit? And the world goes... hurray for "doctor false cheat."[28]

That is idolatry. Idolatry is *not* the Will of God. It is the radical opposite.

Nothing is more uncomfortable for a patient with respiratory difficulties than being proned, forced to lie face down, the diaphragm compressed, nares, nasal passages obstructed.

---

[28] My own parody of Fauci

As a child with chronic, recurrent, severe respiratory conditions, I could only breathe and sleep sitting upright. Face down would be agony and end in suffocation!

At the age of eleven I correctly diagnosed the underlying factor for my recurrent pleuro-pneumonias, etc., but was dismissed with patronising amusement by my lovable but incompetent GP. He would puff on his pipe in my room and say, "call if she gets any worse," and then went on to be appointed Dean of Medicine at Trinity College.

How much worse did it have to get!

And then the psyches – "why do you *want* to be sick..." SMH! So joyful spending weeks in bed, with only books for company, books read with sore and burning eyes!

I correctly diagnosed the status of two relatives to another former Dean of Medicine at Trinity, now in Canada, "printing 3D human brains." Unlike American MDs, he took over their cases without referring back to me.

They died a year later, under orthodox treatment. Where is the logic in poisoning a defenseless, often toxic immune system?

He also did not tell me that one of my brother's was dying. *For three years.*

My treatment would not require a year on a morphine drip – as there was no evidence of pain, btw; nor irradiation, for a condition that the Homeopath would treat oh so gently, and effectively. Requires skill, not the Health Food Store *reductio ad absurdam* of "this for this and that for that..."

Totality of symptoms, must be carefully gathered, minutely assessed, then followed very carefully, matched to the correct, deeply researched remedy and followed closely.

Pre my discovery of Homeopathy, my agonising back pain was treated with unlimited high potency pain killers and the admonition "come back if it gets any worse."

I was a teenager wondering "how much worse must it get…" To parody the late, great Lewis Carroll[29] "to what degree of "worseness" must this worse and worser become!"

The backless "bar stools" in the school's basement science laboratory were the worst. And so I ended up with aspirin poisoning. It's a miracle that I survived Irish Medicine.

And so, when it came time to enter Med School, I said to myself: "This doesn't work" and instead, entered Math Physics, aka "rocket science," in honor of and appreciation for Dr. Alan Gregg, of Oxford and Trinity College Dublin, who gave me a great love for Physics.

And great love for his wife Letty (Letitia) and son John, now also a professor at Oxford. The weekly lesson and gourmet Cordon Bleu dinner from Letty, a brilliant woman and champion of excellence in academia as well as her home and family, all gave me something to look forward to every week.

My mother, Phyllis Kellman Kelleher, barely spoke to me during my entire life, and saw me as a rival to her favorites, my sister Maureen and brother Dermot.

Ironic since she was also from a large family and should have understood that "cohesiveness counts."

She missed her siblings terribly but never openly expressed that loss and refused every opportunity to return. I conjecture that Maureen and Dermot were their "replacements."

---

[29] Mathematician and author of Alice in Wonderland, etc.

So, a life of undiagnosed and improperly managed pain and recurrent infections, septicemia, and severe respiratory illness, spent mostly alone in a room on the top floor with a distant view of the Irish "snot green"[30] sea!

And then I discovered Homeopathy! Back pain gone – still a vulnerability after years of maltreatment, but a viable lifestyle awaited me. I could make appointments with confidence.

Unlike American MDS graduating in the ethical era of the *de rigeur* Hippocratic oath, my brother did not return to confer with me about our parents, nor did this paragon of Medicine even advise me that he had begun to treat them, that my father had died after suffering from chemo radiation for... porphyria... and I do believe that he had called out for me on his death bed. Neither did they tell me that my baby brother   was dying – over a three year period.

He was single and prosperous. His shirts were exquisite. He was also gentle and kind, but was "only" an acoustical engineer from Jaguar and high end motors in England

My other deceased baby brother ran the mainframe computers for England's British Telecom. Two out of four of the baby brothers whom I cared for and from whom I was abruptly separated died in their forties. I wonder if the abrupt separation from their "mother" and suppression of forbidden grief, plus absence of care and feeding impacted on their fragile childhood constitutions, shortening their life spans.

Yet such was the "power" of the "MD" / GP "doktah" status for which the first male was being groomed, that the four younger sons and most brilliant daughter had to be sacrificed.

---

[30] James Joyce, Ulysses again...the "snot green sea!"

Both parents died within two years of my diagnostic information to my brother: 18 months on radiation for my father and a year on morphine for my mother.

I have no doubt that under my care the outcome would have better, kinder, healthier and the life-span longer, and, again, healthier and more productive.

However, my father, brilliant though he was, was still a "test tube" scientist, and so related better and succumbed to his son, the pharma-doc, now ghoulishly "printing human brains" in BCU, Vancouver, Canada! After all his wife made him give up his seat by the fire for her favorite son!

The Classical, Hahnemannian Homeopath is light years ahead of that.

While the Pharma / "health care" industry has stolen much from the Homeopaths, they cannot begin to address the level of authentic scientific analysis, observational skills and "syntheism" with which we diagnose and treat our patients.

"Syntheism" is my word for working *with* the systems placed in the human person by the Creator, each system working independently, but in complete co-operation and harmony with all created systems. Except under duress.

There were inheritance issues as well, which I did not fight, but, basically, being the genius of an extended family comprising many "pedestrian" MDs, with connections to the *harma industry, via research grants, etc., is a bit like being a lamb surrounded by starving, angry jackals.

An existential threat! Mutual — because if the public knew the beauty, power and authority and authentic science of Homeopathy, the *harmaceutical industry would collapse by, say, 75%.

And many hospitals would close – for all the right reasons.

You would not have hundreds of dancing nurses, technicians and MDS ready and willing to throw a sick person on his face, intubate and cut out his or her organs. The truth will out!

Sadly there will always be a need for "heroic medicine" as Homeopaths refer to a system requiring heroism on the part of its patients, and the 25% residual pharmacopeia can be useful in extreme accidents and desperate procedures.

There is a lesson there to, for parents "playing favorites." Entitlement leads to arrogance thence to indifference, thence to callousness.

The "discarded" children can make a choice: focus on anger and its sidekick, vengeance, the "dish best served cold," or focus on compassion and kindness. I had wonderful role models in my teachers in England and the Greggs.

My father, Derry Kelleher, was concerned, but for abstract humanity.

He had a sense of Justice. Indeed that was the title of his imprint, as he started to self-publish under "Justice Books."

However, like most lefties he could not see, recognise, nor wish to face the injustice that was occurring in his own home, right under his nose. Like many lefties, he married into a wealthy family.

My great grandfather was the embroiderer royal and couturier to Queen Victoria.

His sudden, great, prestigious appointment and the strange likeness of my mother to Queen Elizabeth suggests that he may have also provided other services.

After all, Prince Albert and Queen Victoria were first cousins, which did not bode well for future offspring.

Yes, until the Homeopaths were called in to treat Queen Victoria and her children, the children of Victoria and Albert were born with serious congenital anomalies, aka birth defects.

So did the Homeopaths correct the genetic anomalies directly – as we can, so gently and effectively - or did they recommend the use of surrogates?

And was one of them my great grandfather?

Either way, Victoria's ensuing offspring survived and assumed thrones and positions of authority all across Europe.

And the Homeopaths were awarded a unique Royal Charter.

Which King Charles III amended to include all alternative protocols, including those untested, untried and unproven.

And now the NHS claims there is "no proof for the efficacy of Homeopathy."

Balderdash!

Someone was **paid off.**

Our Hospitals had superior survival rates in epidemics, in trauma, in infant survival rates, in mental health, in lowered to ZERO incidents or attempted suicides in prisons or mental hospitals run by Homeopaths – Middletown Hospital, NY, for example, under the famous Dr. Allen.

GSK-Pfizer and cohorts moved into PA because it had become a central hub of Homeopathic expertise and research. The AMA was set up by Rockefeller to suppress us. Our Hospitals were taken over, and our records hidden or destroyed.

That was the primary purpose of the takeovers – to *hide the proof of Homeopathy's extraordinary superiority!!!*

Extraordinary, until you consider the Gamiliel Principle: If it is of God it will prevail.

We have prevailed and will continue to so do, as long as the Almighty so desires.

I was determined to study "nuclear medicine," until a flu shot paralysed me at the age of 15, and I completely lost faith in *harma medicine.

And now, I am an expert in *sub molecular "medicine" aka* **Homeopathy!**

Ironically, it was *harma's own product that **turned the lights on for me.**

God is The Word. The Logos, the Alpha and the Omega...The First Word and the LAST!

Amen!

CHAPTER 22 – The China Syndrome

If multiple, well founded reports are correct, and at this point, there is no reason to doubt, the methods used for "treating" "Covid" are the *identical* methods used for removing organs from living political prisoners in China.

Painful as it may be to consider, if the USA is sending its meat to China to be processed, *what exactly, is China sending back?*

"Back when," the NY Times featured an article on a Chinese **pediatrician** enjoying **a fetal "won ton" soup** or *variation thereof.*

In the media trade that sort of article was equated with "flying a kite," i.e., launching and seeing if it soars.

There may have been a huge backlash because there were no further reports nor public response that I knew of.

However, the more recent news that American meats are shipped to China for rendering does fill me with alarm.

So why was a freighter filled with the bodies of Americans found in the wreckage of a Chinese freighter off the shores of NYS almost a decade ago, without any official report from news, police or Federal agency?

Were they homeless or just members of New York's "single person "families?""

Having sold all our manufacturing industries to China are we now so deeply in debt from buying back our products that we sell the bodies of our poor to them? *For what purpose?*

Were they "hoovered" up from the streets, put in a "dying room" aka negligent or no care "unit" and left to rot and die or killed?

Street sleeper with apparent gangrene, greenish black discoloration of lower limbs BEGGED not to go to hospital.

That is, did they die in hospital with no person to stand by, question the deletion or insertion of DNRs[31] or other unsigned, unapproved documents into the files of vulnerable and unprotected patients?

If those spokespersons for the Church are ignorant of those methods used, then they are at fault for not keeping up with the techniques used in these vile institutions by these ghoulish surgeons, licensed and determined to kill.

And, of course, the "transplant team" more often comes from *outside* the hospital, i.e., is *contracted* rather than employed, to limit liability.

Yes, credit to good surgeons and caring hospitals where credit is due, but these are not targets of my concern and they appear to be very rare creatures indeed!

Sad to say, too many of the better physicians, the "Hippocratic Oath" generation of Physicians who put their patients first, and did not push the mRNA bioweapon and who were personally known to me, have retired or been coerced into retirement during Covid.

Like them or not, and I like many, because we share the same impulse to relieve suffering, the desire to relieve suffering is vocational, a calling, and is different in effect and attitude from the socially aspirant "technicians" graduating from today's Medical Schools, and, in the USA at least, forced to do 90 hour shifts during internship, and if not completely burned out at the conclusion, thence to "Residency" and Boards.

---

[31] DNR is a "Do Not Resuscitate" order signed by patients or family when patient is admitted into hospital. It is fraught with legal uncertainties.

"Doc Martin" syndrome. Automatons without compassion.

By which time, pulling out the prescription pad and signing it becomes reflexive, or perhaps, even dissociative.

One foreign born cardiac specialist admitted that when a patient is referred to them, as a last resort, they simply go through the list of medicines already prescribed, and then write the ones not yet taken.

Or in experimental mode!

Academia in collusion with pHARMa-kopeia?

There's a surprise!

Free gifts, top class stethescopes, pens, notepads, and Heaven knows what else – such as invitations to "seminars," well "oiled" cocktail parties ensued by early lecture, with unattainable and highly distracting coffee wafting through the lecture hall or ballroom of a four or five star hotel...

Academies were founded by Catholic monks, particularly Celtic monks, gifted in art, scripture, literature, music and law.

They were environmentalists, draining swamps, planting eucalyptus trees (Bologna) to deter the influx of mosquitos, and constructing enduring buildings, with shade, warmth and shelter.

They grew their own food, raised sheep and milk cows, and followed the Creator's plan in developing sustainable self-sufficiency.

They were brilliant herbalists, dedicated, selfless men, who, at risk of their own lives, provided sanctuary for the wounded, the falsely accused, those at risk of their lives, and orphans.

Yes, corruption took over from time to time, wartime conditions stressing all aspects of daily life, secular and religions. Corruption was always overthrown, although the battle against corruption continues to rage - even in this day and age of intense secularism.

CHAPTER 23 -   Doctrine of Similars

The monks studied the plants intently, trying to understand the Creator's intent for each plant, and which properties were unique to a particular plant.

They discovered the "Doctrine of Similars," that is, that the phyto healers were coded according to the organs to which they would be of greatest benefit and for which they were created.

Purple, for the heart. Foxglove, aka Digitalis!

Yellow, for the liver. Buttercup, and the phenomenal dandelion, root and leaf...leaf cleansing, root healing.

Red Clover – anti-inflammatory, decongestant...

Peppermint, White or pale pink "worm" shaped flower: anti-helminthic... parasite cleanser!

And so on.

A personal observation – is that the more "common" and ubiquitous the plant, that is with the status of "weed," the greater its power to heal, and its both general and specific applications.

And the greater the power of that plant, aka a humble "weed," the more the Creator hides it in plain sight!

Keeping out of the way of the condescending and profiteering pHARMaceutical industries.

 "What does He know! He's only the carpenter's son!"[32]

I now leave the herbs to our blessed herbalists...

---

[32] Biblical reference to pharisaical snobbery.

CHAPTER 24 – Infertility 2

There are many good reasons why Homeopaths should not reveal the name of the remedy prescribed.

"Linguistic over-ride" is one. It is a new 21st century term for what used to be known as "instinct," e.g., the sudden urge to turn off the main road and take a different route home…which, if followed, leads to safety, but which, if ignored, leads to a mile long traffic jam due to some terrible accident on a usually safe highway.

Some call it Divine Inspiration, the whisper of angels, and or the power of the unconscious mind or "super conscious."

Whatever the dynamic, our remedies work best if left to said "superconscious," "linguistic over-ride," or "intelligence" of the immune system.

Besides that, some of our genotypes are highly intelligent "ferrets" determined to follow every nano system, and in that way, actually *over –ride the immune system's cellular intelligence*[33] *and sabotage their own recovery.*

This genotype predictably announces at follow up appointments that "nothing has changed." At which time, our meticulous notes become vital as we can then "tick off" a multitude of symptoms that did respond to the Homeopathic similar!

Aforesaid "genotype" arrives with copious notes, records, tests, etc.

We prefer a relaxed, low intensity setting, to relax our beloved patients and encourage them to describe their systems in whichever order they choose, which sequence is more

---

[33] "Cellular Intelligence" – expression alien to the allopaths or *harmaceutical industry.

instructive to us than a hard drive filled with lab work. Of course that has its place, but is secondary to the information provided directly by our patient!

The worst danger in divulging the names of the prescribed remedy is that Big Pharma will grab it, promote it and destroy it, as they did with St. John's Wort, promoting it as a cure all for depression. It is an extraordinary Gift to humanity, but not as a liver remedy.

Homeopathists and the "acupuncture of the *superior doctor*" concur in considering the liver as the primary seat of depression. Sorry, shrinks!

More on that later, but if anything proves the foresight of the Founding Fathers of Homeopathy, it is that Rule. Do not divulge!

In these harrowed times, however, I have been obliged – most unwillingly – to skirt that rule, as well as another vital rule, and that is not to treat patients already under medication.

*It appears that, post 9/11 90% of civilisation is on some form of Prescription medication, and, as one Rx leads to side effects and ten more Rxs, and the Health Authorities, aided, abetted, funded, sponsored, "fed, walked and watered" by Big *harma, have now changed the parameters or "paradigms" for certain* **chronic** *diseases such as diabetes, I know have to antidote the meds and dance around the symptoms in order to determine with are autochtonous and which are iatrogenic.*

That is which are natural or intrinsic to the patient and which are caused by the *harma meds!

Non-disclosure of name of other meds by patient.

Many reasons for that – the most vital one, is that the results will not be as outstanding, and the remedies may have to be repeated as the prescription pHARMa meds often antidote the carefully prescribed Homeopathics.

And when a patient is on Oxycontin and does not advise the Homeopath accordingly, treatment will be incredibly frustrating.

An expert Homeopath has a fair idea of the sequences of recovery, depending on case and remedy provided, and so when the patient remains *"status quo"* long after treatment and anticipated onset of recovery, early signs or complete recovery, then the truth is revealed.

Nothing shuts down the immune system and the cerebro-spinal circuits like neuro toxins, sometimes handed out like candy at Christmas to "heart sink"[34] patients by the allopaths or pHARMa docs.

Homeopaths have methods to "clean" or detox a compromised system, but where pregnancy is desired, and a patient has been on strong medications, it is best to allow six months for the body to clear residual toxins before starting to consider conceiving a beautiful baby.

Detox includes anti-doting hormones and medicinal herbals.

It is hard to believe that OB-GYNs prescribed equine estrogen to menopausal women. Equine cell replication is 40 times the rate of humans!!!

Analogous to traumatising delicate breast tissue prior to irradiating by mammogram!

So, if fertility is an issue or a last chance baby is longed for, clear the system of invasive hormones and substances.

---

[34] "Heartsink" is an allopath's term for the patient who arrives with multiple symptoms, is chronically ill, and, understandably, dissatisfied. Homeopaths LOVE complex cases!

If you are overweight, start exercising.

If you are underweight, allow yourself a few extra pounds.

If you are addicted to any substance, advise your Homeopath.

If you are using contraceptives or have a history of abortion, advise your Homeopath.

If you are using or have used in vitro, advise your Homeopath.

If you are using or have tried the NFP method, with no conception or conception followed by miscarriage, also advise your Homeopath.

If you have undergone radiation, also advise your Homeopath.

If you are in an abusive relationship, advise your Homeopath.

Any and all information is completely confidential and is directed to understanding and removing any and all impediments to helping you arrive at optimum health so that you may conceive and safely carry a sweet and beautiful baby to term without intrusive and ignominious practice and further harm to your person.

Or questions are "scientific," not judgmental, and are designed to understand the *causa radica* of infertility and treat according to the **totality of symptoms.**

Every new birth is an occasion of great joy.

CHAPTER 26 – Infertility 3

The Homeopath's approach.

No, you don't go to the Health Food Store and look at the one symptom printed on Boiron's "Blue tubes!"

We consider the patient's general physical appearance and health.

We then ask a lot of questions, including genetic heritage.

Some are the same as the "ghoul school." Most appear abstruse and irrelevant.

And are anything but.

Of all the factors imported from post Maoist China, we bring the "acupuncture of the inferior doctor."

Not the unusual and time proven "exotic" skills of the "superior doctor."

For example....

...For the comfort of the patient and to identify any unexpected or covert factors, I take the Oriental pulses, mentioned in a previous chapter.[35] There are 14, most relevant to an individual organ, others to general health and metabolism.

The pace of the pulse is one thing; the quality and tenor completely different, and, in practice, incredibly informative.

But like the digits of the violinist, sensitivity and practice are essential.

They "beat" New York Hospital's Emergency Room tests in identifying the source of my young neighbour's pain!

---

[35] Homeopathy and Celibacy

Homeopathy functions brilliantly with a different skillset, most analysis and comparative analyses, but it can be comforting to the patient to know the sources of pain or illness, or as the Homeopaths said it first, the *causa radica,* that is, root cause.

Especially in chronicity when patients are often happy when the "outer layer" of symptoms is removed, but more is required to prevent the return of any and all symptoms, and to facilitate full recovery and maximum health.

It is always necessary to ask about pregnancies, whatever the motivating concern for the initial consult.

Birth injury, birth fatigue, nutritional deficiencies, infection, chronic illness, anemias, lack of support and shred tasks can deeply affect the general health and metabolism of a mother, especially a single mother.

These can drastically affect not only the ability to conceive but the ability to carry a child to term.

A previous abortion can be devastating, mentally, emotionally, physically.

One young woman answered negatively: "No, no pregnancies," then suddenly started to clutch her abdomen as if something was churning within.

"Yes" "she said, "late term," and ran out of the consulting room before I could tell her about Project Rachel and other resources for PAS.

Her baby's desperate struggle for survival were imprinted in her biological memory.

I have met teenagers, forced to have as many as four abortions – forced by their own mothers... desperate to carry their child to term but too terrified of their own mothers to avail of the many 'rescues" offered by Pro Life Groups.

Two of the coerced young women, were, in fact, in their early twenties, but raised in cults.

One was used in rituals from the age of eight, ended up institutionalised for years, was then able to start over, but with the "killer grandmother" living nearby she became pregnant again, crying that she wanted her baby, aborted again and back to the psychiatric residences, more than likely for the rest of her life.

Her apartment was spotless, sterile, reflecting her life.

Women with Post Abortion Syndrome are nine times as likely to attempt suicide as women with no history of abortion.

But back to LIFE.

Repairing the emotional scars of abortion. This must be considered with utmost compassion and sensitivity.

Homeopaths have remedies that can release suppressed emotions, but they must not be handled by amateurs.

A beloved long term "patient" asked why I only used a certain remedy in the lower potencies, i.e., the 30c, and I provided the above answer.

"But my brother took a 1M – high potency – and had no problems with it."

What were his symptoms?

They were physical, digestive and diet related with a somewhat "stoic" personality.

Now the 1M also addressed emotional trauma, very deeply, otherwise the release of suppressed pain may overwhelm. It is therefore considered only where there is a very strong support system, and patient is advised of potentially intense reaction and to have friends and comfort nearby.

The 30c may be repeated, gently over time. The 1M, usually just one dose, one time only.

Initial consult:

To be considered:

Constitution, aka genomic heritage.

"Indigenous" physical and emotional dynamics.

Acquired physical and emotional dynamics.

Personality – general

Personality – specific, e.g., type A, type B, etc?

Physical Appearance

Ethnicity

Diet and Nutrition

Preferred foods

Dietary aversions

Lifestyle

General symptoms

Specific Symptoms

Peculiar symptoms

The Homeopath does *not* judge, does *not* make formal diagnoses. Though we understand the language of the pHARMa physicians, we file it as interesting, do not dismiss it outright, but we have our own, superior methodology for interpreting and understanding the myriad metabolic disorders that affect the human person, along with specific psychological, emotional and traumatic affects and. Implications, *and, of course, extrinsic factors*.

Extrinsic factors would include inadequate living conditions, toxic work environments, chem-trails, bombs, war zones, violent crimes, etc.

However, prior abortion seems to increasingly factor in the incidence of low fertility and spontaneous miscarriage.

Dilation and "curettage" is where the "green, stiff" sphincters of the "unripe" protective cervix are forced open.

Ever force a, say, brachial upper arm muscle to hold weights beyond its capacity for a prolonged period?

Rupture, tear, sprain… even hairline fracture of the underling bone can follow and be all but impossible to repair.

The cervix forced open unnaturally, cannot close naturally.

This inevitably leads to infection, unmodulated periods and the inability to carry a baby to term.

Often surgery is required.

The Homeopath can do a certain amount, depending on the damage, using the most appropriate trauma remedies, but closing a cervix ruptured after a late term abortion is all but impossible without surgery.

Neuro surgeons at London's 'Hospital for Special Surgery' would ask us to pre and post treat their surgical patients as they would then recover more rapidly, with zero infections.

Homeopathy can be used diagnostically as well

For example, a beautiful young woman was having difficulty conceiving a second child. She was in good health and a very kind an considerate person. I could not understand why her symptoms pointed to a potential (remedy) that was associated with angry, resentful women.

However, the symptom picture concurred in every other way, and so I prescribed the indicated remedy and two months later, she was pregnant.

 And yes, there was significant cause for that remedy, though with her good nature the emotional symptoms were contained and still quite healthy. Prolonged imposed stress.

Emotional stress such as grief or loss due to location displacement can deeply disrupt the endocrinal system.

Prolonged grief, or just not having needs met as a child can lead to withdrawal and introversion.

Monosyllables, polite but curt or abbreviated answers combined with physical symptoms, also pointing to trauma, retention, sadness, can quickly be resolved by a certain remedy, one which actually causes sterility in its material form.

CHAPTER 27 - Abortion and Infertility

There are many causes of infertility, from injury, to medication, to congenital or inherited conditions, to fibroids, stress related symptoms, prolonged use of hormones or contraceptives, poor diet, abortifacients, malnutrition, impaired absorption; environmental hazards, chemo-radiation, chemical warfare, the atomic – nuclear bombs of Hiroshima and Nahasaki…prior abortions and it is an absolute miracle that any child or Gen X,Y,Z, Millennium, Alpha, Beta, Boomer or even post Boomer has survived!

Due to the prevalence of abortion in the USA, the "sighting" of a baby or child is now a rare event!

No children playing in their yards; no children scooting or skating on the streets…

I can just imagine the shock and horror of the liberal pro-abortionists at the very idea of streets filled with happy, laughing, naughty children, with or without their parent - or in self-protective groups…

Odd how many child abusers are pro abortion!

The deranged want children to be slaughtered *in utero,* to remain invisible, out of sight, once their bloodied bodies are disposed of, trashed, dismembered for "spare parts," or sold to cosmetic corporations for "skin care" or other "beauty" products.

Kuru Kuru, a motor neuron disease, aka "Mad Cow" Disease is a product of cannibalism, which can also be a factor where trans-dermal absorption is involved as in skin care products.

Major skin care producers fail to answer a simple question: Is aborted baby tissue of any kind used in skin care products… SILENCE upon SILENCE.

For those women coerced into abortion, there is hope and support. Project Rachel is profoundly healing according to persons benefiting from their retreats, and there are other resources to assist with the emotional and spiritual aspects, which have often affected the ability of a woman to bring a child to term after a previous abortion. The methods used to terminate a pregnancy, that is, murder a baby *in utero* or during partial birth are crying out to the Heavens for justice.

During pregnancy the cervix serves as a "fortress," stiff, closed, and impenetrable. In colloquial terminology – "green," unripe.

At the time of natural delivery, the longitudinal muscles soften, the cervix widens, the mucus plug protecting the baby from infection, etc., is released and *natural labor commences.*

This allows for an easier delivery, and faster recovery.

Inductions may be necessary but rare; however, they are overused, often with the intention of deliberately harming both mother and child.[36]

The difference between Home Birth and "Normal" Hospital Birth is about $2,000. The difference between "Normal Hospital Birth" and Induction is about $10,000. The difference between induction and caesarian is $30,000 - $50,000. Now, factor in damage to mother and baby and add another $50k to the Caeserian!

Before you rant and rail here's a relevant quote from one of the leading protagonists of Roe v Wade: Dr. Bernard Nathanson, RIP. "Medicine is a business."

Up to 1973 we thought of it as a vocation, a calling! Nathanson recanted became a Catholic. He also gave us the following line:

---

[36] https://www.sarawickham.com/research-updates/induction-increases-caesarean/

"It is hard to convince yourself that you are not taking human life when you are ***throwing little arms and legs into a bucket.***

"What do you mean by "little arms and legs?"" asked a young neighbour who was bragging about serving as a "Deathscort."[37]

"Don't you know what you are supporting and promoting?" I replied, and proceeded to enlighten her.

The Chemicals used in inducing what is usually *premature labour* are the same as those used in late term abortions. The artificially induced contractions are more intense and prolonged, than natural labor with its periodic rest intervals. The mother can seize mid contraction, the taut muscles compressing her baby's head, causing possible damage to the tender tissues of the brain.

It is certainly highly traumatic and potentially FATAL.

I know of one baby who would start screaming if required to go into elevators or if he heard a trolly.

Because they resonated with the memories of the hospital and his horrific and avoidable trauma.

The majority of women bullied, repeat *bullied* into inductions are "nullipara," giving birth to their first baby, and I would wager, they would mostly be single mothers.

I also wager that a certain percentage are told that their baby did not survive and/or would need disability care for the rest of his or her sweet life.

---

[37] "Deathscort:"Person who steers pregnant women into abortuaries, and away from those "terrible" pro Lifers who try to help her and save her baby's life.

It is also likely that the babies who did "not survive" were being used for "organ donations," no doubt with the consent of a shocked, traumatised, grieving, over medicated mother!

That mother will not be informed that her baby is lying on a tray in a surgical unit, writhing in agony as his or her organs are removed, one by one and expedited to another state for transplant.

All the "wonderful" techniques we learn from Communist China!

That human kind could descend to such cruelty, sadism and viciousness, is incomprehensible without two factors.

The insidiousness of syphilis…and its destruction of the meninges of the human brain.

The most sadistic leaders of the world suffered from syphilis, either actively acquired or hereditary.

With the poor sanitation of previous centuries it was a constant hazard – promiscuity not required! This led to "lead" and mercury poisoning, other contributors to the mental illness of worlds driven by greed and corruption.

Henry VIII, Elizabeth I, Hitler, Mao and probably Genghis Khan, Attila the Hun, and a person misnamed as a "prophet" were all syphilitic. Henry VIII murdered his wives, transmitted syphilis to his daughter, Elizabeth the First, causing her to be infertile, and in order to cover that up, she re-identified as "The Virgin Queen," a usurpation of the title of the beloved Mary of Nazareth, aka Queen of Heaven, and murdered every Catholic "guilty" of hyperdulia, not worship, but mega respect for Mary, the Mother of Christ our Savior.

Centuries later, many Protestants are still imprinted with fear of respecting the Mother of Jesus.

Just as the Irish still dance with their hands held rigidly by their sides – a style brought from Spain by Elizabeth 1 of England - to teach the Irish self discipline!

"How's that working, then!" Sez the Irish!

Elizabeth I never married because she could not carry a child, and it is likely that she could not conceive.

In those centuries there was some medical intelligence or cohesion, at least where syphilis was concerned.

However, if a woman was infertile, it was assumed that "she bin' to the witch," or was, herself a "witch."

That is, an **abortionist.**

Abortionists moved into, or more commonly, just outside a village, and the birth rate moved out! Methods used were herbal, phyto toxins, which I shall not disclose here.

If someone wishes to avail of abortifacient phyto toxins they will have to seek elsewhere. Abuse of said toxins can be lethal.

Some were already in use by registered doctors to induce the little bodies of babies who died *in utero,* by natural causes or accidental exposure to toxins.[vi]

Others may have been used by GPs/internists acting as covert abortionists. The "private surgery" abortions listed as "miscarriage."

One of said phyto toxins being the rye fungus **ergot.** [38]

However, as ergot is terrifyingly toxic, with effects such as vaso constrictions leading to limitations on blood flow, thereby to gangrene, thereby to amputations, etc., there is little risk of it

---

[38]https://www.fs.usda.gov/wildflowers/ethnobotany/Mind_and_Spirit /ergot.shtml

being used by non-professionals, who being sociopathic or psychopathic and sadistically inclined, seem to prefer dismemberment or surgical butchery.

We can probably antidote the effects of ergot or the morning after pill, but it would take a team of surgeons to repair the effects of the infamous "coat hanger" for example!!!

Interestingly, in the USDA link below, *it is not described as an abortiacient, but as the source of Lysergic Acid, aka LSD!*

Hence the insanity!

Source, again, the "satanists!" Destroyers of Life.

The fungus is partial to rye, a grain used in making bread and popular in Northern Europe and flourished in a particularly wet growing season leading to severe injury and deaths in the Franco-German areas of the Holy Roman Empire and the dissolution of the Empire.

God does not seek our destruction or death. Perhaps absolute power corrupted absolutely and the Romans forgot to be holy and were then called to conversion and repentance.

That is a question, not a statement. Theology is not my area of expertise, although the care and cure of the ill are close and blessed "cousins!"

However, it does "beg the question" of the challenges facing the Catholic Church today with so few prelates speaking openly against abortion, and those who do, being chastised and punished.

It "begs the question" of the failure to fully comprehend the self-perpetuating effects of "interrupting" Creation by murdering the offspring of Catholic and non-Catholic unions, and the extreme but logical consequences of slashing and dismembering a helpless but GIFTED wee baby, which consequences being the **slashing and dismembering** of the human family, community, parish, society, and **deposit of Faith.**

Every wee baby is unique and irreplaceable. Each and every baby brings GIFTS into the world, the greatest of these being the **unconditional** LOVE of God, manifested in the sweet smile and gentle caress of the infant.

Each baby comes with a GIFT and a Challenge. *Sometimes the Challenge is the true Gift, and the Gift turns out to be the Challenge.* My "genius" made enemies: my illness made me a Homeopath, able to help many, thank God!

In my own life, my Gifts were considered exceptional and extraordinary and yes, they inspired kindness in some quarters, notably my English teachers, Mr. Mott and Mrs. Simmonds of Hampshire, UK, but they also inspired pathological jealousy in my own family and outrage as the "English girl" from the upper Mid family took scholarships from poorer Irish country lads. Not complaining, just analysing. It was nice to fast track languages and music.

The Challenge was ill health, a rare, undiagnosed anemia which kept me bedridden for much of my childhood and teen years. Again, the Hampshire, UK country doctors were great. Insofar as England's National Health didn't cover costly diagnostics, the prescriptions of Dandelion and Burdock were incredibly restorative, and probably led to my pursuit of Homeopathy.

I was about to enter ordinary Medical School but took a long walk around the Greystones sea coast and left with the realisation that I would be spending another 7 years with my rejecting mother and **IT DIDN'T WORK!**

My GP in Ireland was lovable, but hopeless and became the Dean of Medicine at Trinity College, followed by my brother, equally hapless as a diagnostician, and now, as I predicted, a research scientist printing 3D Human Brains.

Sadly, I correctly diagnosed both parents' conditions and, regrettably, advised him accordingly.

They were both dead within two years – closer to one!!!

My honest opinion now, is that those men who ride the garbage trucks and are not considered "gifted" enough for University or Medical School, actually do more for Public Health than all the Pharmaceutical Corporations, Harvard Med, U Penn, UNC., etc., combined!

The best medical doctors with whom I am acquainted in the USA were all trained in Italy.

Until Fauci hooked up with Draghi compassion was never a crime in Italy.

CHAPTER 28 - Racism In Medicine.

The galloping increase in motor neuron degenerative disease in white populations in the USA[39] and Europe[40] since the inception and promotion of "low cholesterol" and other fad diets is staggering.

It has doubled in under two decades! Due to, er, "longevity," some environmental factors, *but no mention is ever made of the toxicity of the "vaccine" injuries, nor of the susceptibility of the Northern, "Viking" populations to a number of rare anemias.*

Nor do they mention the probability of covert" "kuru kuru" or motor neuron cannibal disease through digestion or transdermal absorption of pre-natal human tissue from the use of aborted baby body parts in cosmetics and food products.

Neurological disorders are now the leading source of disability in the world, and Parkinson's disease is the fastest growing of these disorders. "As the population ages and life expectancy increases, the number of individuals with Parkinson's disease will continue to increase as well as the duration of the disease, leading to more patients with advanced Parkinson's disease."

Neurological disorders are now the leading source of disability in the world, and Parkinson's disease is the fastest growing of these disorders.

And mass "vaccination" of mulltiple pathogens is the most aggressively promoted treatment...

Then again, the Lancet paper is funded by the... drumroll – Bill and Melinda Gates Foundation...[41] notorious for their

---

39 w.ncbi.nim.nih.gov/parkinsons
40 WHO – prevalence of Parkinsons
41 https://www.thelancet.com/journals/laneur/article/PIIS1474-4422%2818%2930295-3/fulltext

promotion of toxic and lethal vaccination - so notorious, in fact that the Government of India imposed a death sentence on Gates *in absentia.*

Ketogenic deserves a special mention, producing the same symptoms as starvation, or drinking nail polish remover, but the greater culprits, "accessories after the fact of vaccines" are the "low cholesterol" and vegan diets.

While, I am 100% behind free will in choice of diet, health care, etc., it is hardly an authentic "choice" if the appropriate and relevant information and risks are not disclosed.

Why "Racism?"

Heritage Europeans, particularly of the Northern, Viking realms are particularly susceptible to the malabsorption of Vitamin B12, a substance vital to the development of healthy red blood cells and central nervous system.

"Vitamin" seems to be an understatement in regards to the extraordinary power and influence of metho or cyano-cobalamin, and an inappropriate category for a substance that holds such power over LIFE AND DEATH and is the determining factor whether a life will be healthy and productive one, or one of constant sickness, disappointment, fragility, low stamina, weakness, chronic pain, slow healing, etc.

Elizabeth Barrett Browning, Emily Dickinson, Bronte Sisters and Brother, Jane Austen, and other fragile geniuses, all manifest the signs and symptoms of prolonged B12 deficiency.

To deprive persons of Northern European Heritage of B12 is a crime crying out to Heaven for punishment.

And yet our children are seldom tested, and it is a battle royal to persuade the allopaths to test an adult with glaringly obvious symptoms for B12 deficiency.

How many miscarriages could have been avoided had appropriate tests been done.

Sickle cell tests are routine for black African American children in the USA so I have to ask the question, in conjunction with other observations: Is there a covert program of genocide of the white, Aryan, Euro Christian peoples.

You know, the ones who invented cars, running water, central heating, socks, shoes, windows, doors, books, libraries, schools, Universities, printing presses, computers, math, astronomy, fine art, fridges, violins, pianos, organs, jets... that sort of thing...

Is it that the rest of the world who didn't make such inventions, covet what we have, and will destroy us through attritional genocide, or planned genocide.

Because I cannot fathom any other logical reason for withholding Vitamin B12 from the productive and protective members of the human race.

Other than the intention to maximise suffering and thereby maximise profit from hazardous meds and extreme procedures.

Best sources of B12: Beef, calves or beef liver (!!!) Venison, Egg yolk, Salmon, etc.

These are all pro-scribed, i.e., discouraged by the low cholesterol diet.

The low cholesterol diets are pre-scribed , i.e., ordered by the *harma docs, allopaths, etc., and directed at the affluent middle class white populations, i.e., those with good insurance!

RACISM AGAIN!

So given that connection, given the susceptibility, vulnerability and incidence of B12 malabsorption, aka *pernicious anemia* in

"Viking" populations, why are children never tested for B12 malabsorption instead of being directed to a shrink who asks *"why do you **want** to be sick?"*

Seriously, what child *wants* to be sick, and can generate the symptoms concommitant to B12 deficiency???

So cruel to a child in pain, gasping for breath!

Do the "Morlochs" [42] understand what chronic or intermittent illness is to a child? That it destroys the social life and self-confidence of a child, leads to isolation, and even parental resentment.

"Why do you want to be shivering but febrile; unable to sit upright, breathe, in constant pain?

*No child could ever **induce such symptoms!***

Before Third World[43] doctors invaded the British Isles, lowered the standard of medicine and hygiene, opened the door to MRSA,[44] the English system used to be more realistic and compassionate – as in GPs [45]prescribing Beef Tea and/or Dandelion and Burdock, an herbal drink high in iron, for the sickly children and adults.

If a case was severe enough for actual lab work, and B12 deficiency, or pernicious anemia or Addisonians was discovered, then the hapless patient would be "blessed" with chopped calves liver injected directly into the glutei.

---

[42] "Morloch" is my nickname for the most aggressive, bullying, incompetent members of a once kindly, albeit backward profession.
[43] *Repeat Third World "doctors" with fake degrees and various levels of competency...*
[44] *In the UK, MRSA was attributed to moslem doctors and nurses refusing to regularly wash hands and sanitise between each consult. IMO the newly sealed windows in hospitals that once insisted on "fresh" air irrespective of weather conditions were another factor.*
[45] *GP: General Practitioner, analogous to "internist."*

May have saved a few lives, marriages, etc., but ouch! Today, B12 is more accessible and "delivery" is easier, more versatile, but primarily used for Sickle Cell and Hollywood's addicts!

CHAPTER 29 – Ageism in Medicine

And now the "grown ups!"

Why are Senior citizens on *low cholesterol* diets immediately Dx'd with "Dementia" or Alzheimers, for having less than eidetic memories?

Why are "low cholesterol," i.e., B12 DEFICIENT, diets prescribed for Senior Citizens at a time when their absorption of this life generating substance is diminishing?

Why are Senior Citizens or older adults Dx'd with Parkinsons and instantly prescribed inimical paralysands such as "Aducanumab"[46] at the first sign of a tremor.

The CDC with differential tests, standardised now for most "check ups" do not reveal quality and size of erythrocytes or red blood cells.

An astute diagnostician might see signs worth investigating in other markers, and request more precise and relevant tests, but most just accept the "markers" made by the lab assistants and assume that all is well: that the RBCs are just fine.

B12 absorption diminishes with age, so why cut primary sources of B12 from the seniors' diet! Unless you want mega funding for Alzheimers!

FIRST DO NO HARM!!!

It's a "numbers" game after all...

"Numbers" aren't always exclusive to ... $$$!

Imagine the absurdity of: "Well, congratulations, your cholesterol is lower, but is that a tremor in your hand?"

---

[46] Aducanumab no longer rx'd for Alzheimers in USA.

"You may have early onset Parkinsonian...we'll give you some pills to offset that..."

"Your blood pressure is high too, we'll put you on, (chuckle, chuckle) some water pills."

"Is there a history of dementia in your family..."

After the terrified patient is overloaded with prescriptions and unaware that their condition can be transformed or cured completely - be it erroneous Alzheimers-Parkinsons Dx/projection or genuine signs and symptoms of chronic B12 deficiency, s/he often goes into a depression "needing" more medication.

*Gold mine for the *harma Docs!*

Parents or grandparents depressed or forgetful? Put them "outside" a 6oz lean steam or calves liver if tolerated, or a quality hamburger.

And if the difference is marked, and your MD / GP still refuses to test for B12 deficiency and provide B12 shots, have "Uncle Luigi" pay a visit.

And a few dozen of his compadres...!

And if there are tremors or stiffness of gait, and no sign of improvement after a few weeks on the B12 injections, then BRING YOUR LOVED ONE TO A HOMEOPATH, STATEM.

THERE IS NO EXCUSE OR JUSTIFICATION FOR THIS GENOCIDAL "MEDICINE FROM HELL!"

CHAPTER 30 - Morality, Criminality and Disease.

For the majority of persons for whom the enjoyment of alcohol is *not* a disease, that is, those who can drink moderately, and are not driven by an impulse to drink themselves into a state of oblivion, it is far too easy to judge the alcoholic as a selfish, out of control, immoderate, immature inebriate and ne'er do well.

Outside of crises and trauma, few of us need to drink to "feel normal."

The alcoholic, however, does not feel normal unless s/he is "outside" a few drinks.

Every addict whom I treated or encountered, be it "legit" overmedicated "pillhead" or convulsing on the street heroin addict, each and every one had an alcoholic within three generations of their family history.

All too often the heritage also includes war, famine, infected water, disease, congested hospitals, homelessness, widowed parents, etc...

Which also leads to malnutrition, compromised immunity, and where morality is also compromised in desperation to feed self or family, serious infection, and consequent epidemics of DNA destroying disease.[47]

The bloodlines of alcoholics often include suggestions or even evidence of the genetic sequence of such infections from which it is plausible to infer that the alcoholic's insatiable desire and appetite for alcohol maybe an instinctual manouevre by a deficient but desperate immune system determined to destroy pathogenic invaders.

The immune system is designed to protect and preserve life!

---

[47] "Mitochondrial Murder?" by Dr. Deirdre McNamara

Again, the Human mind and spirit, compromised by certain diseases, STDs such as syphilis, and the amorality and decadence that too often precedes such infections – warps and degenerates the Human psyche to the most bizarre and terrifying extent.

To be very clear, the majority of persons contracting such STDS are not the amoral decadents, but their **victims.**

As I advised a roomful of employees of the US Dept of State and various medical personnel from the "Alfalfabet" agencies, at a time when young and older homosexual men were dying from AIDS, the promiscuity and / or "party life" of such communities led to multiple opportunistic infections, all treated by anti-biotics with subsequent impairment or even destruction of the autochtonous immune system.

The treatment of AIDS changed after that conference, but I received no credit nor invitation to follow up.

I may also have ended up on Fauci's "hit list." As sabotage of a research project pertaining to paralysis, MRSA and respiratory dependency suggests.

Also vulnerable are **victims** of the consequences of war. Poor sanitation, lack of sanitation, sabotaged or over used water supplies, depleted endocrinal systems, digestive systems barraged by toxins or starved of nutrients or all at once, eliminative systems overwhelmed by toxic food, air, fluids, gases.

An exhibition in the Historical Medical Museum in Vienna, Austria, aka "The Josephus" in Vienna, a historical Medical Museum exquisitely proved Dr. Hahnemann's theory of "Miasmic" transmission.

Now the term "Miasm" became obsolete, perhaps with the assistance of Pharmakopei, the "sorcerors'" medicine, but that is conjecture, and Homeopaths like facts and confirmation.

It is a historic Victorian term, perhaps arising from the smog of London past...but since Hahnemann was a German exiled in Paris for curing too many of his compadre's "incurable" diseases, and since smoky coal was the primary source of winter heating, perhaps Paris was smoggy too.

I understand it this. Each disease has its own, unique, symptom "cluster," but inherited strengths and weakness condition its outcome.

If the annihilation of the toxins is incomplete or the damage to DNA too intense, then the secondary effects are transmitted to the next generation.

For example, the Josephus had photographs of the buboes of syphilis, and thence their "offspring" - the tubers of tuberculosis.

Thence, the tumors of cancer, and beyond that, to warts, eczema, moles, and other dermal manifestations of the amazing Divinely installed *protections explicit to the human immune system, and intrinsic to most mammalian and partly indeed to pescine species.*

Hahnemann: Cure begins from above downward, within outward.

The protection of the Brain, Central Nervous System, and internal organs are paramount.

It is my considered opinion that the buboes, tubercles, tumors, warts, etc., are the "toxic waste dumping sites" of the immune system, set aside until the patient's immune system is sturdy or resilient enough to burn it off, through fever, or to resorb it, gradually, assisted or guided perhaps by Homeopathy, along with change in diet, location or habits.

"Toxic waste" being a simplistic but clarifying description.

Of course, if situated in a position to obstruct respiration or elimination, and such, then surgical removal would be justified.

To the other "growths" may now be added the fibrins aka non haemo clots of the "Covid" mRNA bioweapon, clamped into the veins, arteries, etc., out of the way until the Immune System develops a solution. Sadly, a surge in blood pressure or extreme increase in temperature pulls or pushes it off, into circulation and thence into the tiny vessels of the heart, causing cardiac arrest, now speciously termed "myocarditis," or rather, the secondary effect.

That is more logical than the intensive searches for any site to surgically remove, and in so doing, release toxins, mitochondria, rna and Heaven knows what back into circulations.

<u>20th Century Deceptions in Marriage</u>

Until the atrocity of 9/11 and the internet crashed our belief in a sane world largely run by ethical people, naïve women were often coaxed into marriage with aspiring executives, performers, and such, only to spend a life time worrying where their "husbands" were and obsessing over their appearance in the hope of attracting their "other attracted" spouses who were just using them as a "beard."

That is, they covered their homosexual attractions at a time when executives were required to have wives who could efficiently and charmingly host cocktail parties and were therefore essential to promotion.

Understandably, these abused women turned to the aforesaid cocktails and thence became what was "euphemistically" described as "lushes," despised by their own children, living lives of quiet desperation and "mommy's little helpers."

"Mommy's little helpers" was a euphemistic term for librium, valium, etc., or in Ireland, seroxet handed out like candy by indifferent general practitioners, trying to cram as many patients as possible into their hourly schedules before retiring to the medical version of Sunset Boulevard.

I was polite and collegial until the shamdemic aka Covid.

Virginia Wolf was a lesbian who married a homosexual publisher and committed suicide. They were "beards" for one another, which has its limitations, especially in close note Victorian society.

TS Eliot married a brilliant but fragile poet who "checked herself" into a mental hospital. Eliot had a platonic epistolatory "affair" with another English woman who also ended up in a mental hospital. That and the uniquely English style of "Cats" suggest an extremely dark side of Eliot's character, and that is, the *theft* of his wife's work.

Did these men bring disease home to their wives? What motivated them to destroy the brilliant women who gave them a "safe alibi" and kept them out of prison. Homosexuality was a criminal offense in England until 1967.

However, while it was de-criminalised *de jure,* it was still preferable for ambitious young men climbing a corporate ladder to be married, preferably to attractive young women capable of hosting cocktail parties for associates and clients.

I knew of at least one case where the wife found out when husband returned from a trip abroad to announce that he had acquired AIDS.

She almost lost her mind, started to make the rounds of "Irish" pubs in the USA, declaiming dramatically "My husband has AIDS!" She died young, alone and far from her Irish homeland.

Did those men drive their wives to suicide or insanity with rejection, ridicule, virtual abandonment, or, were the roots of mental illness and stability already in place?

Spielberg and Zuckerberg are proven plagiarists, proven in the American courts and on public record. Spielberg's victim was a female writer of childrens' books. Zuckerberg stole from foreign students in the USA, good natured South American brothers who developed Facebook.

Bill Ghates took established computer programs and modified them. He took established vaccine "science" and intensified it to a lethal degree. His wife was the computer scientist with advanced degrees when he married her after seven years of "courtship."[48]

Musk clones off the name of Tesla. Seems absolutely clueless.

Einstein is reportedly not a mathematician but his wife, Mary Clare was... $E = MC^2$???!

Or $MC = E^2$

That is, does it take a multiple of Mary Clares to equal one Einstein, or a multiple of Einsteins to equal ONE Mary Clare!

It is time to stop worshipping the privately selected, publicly assigned "wunderkinder" and to start looking under the stones, and behind the "wardrobes" and taking a little time to differentiate the "Lions" from the "Witches!"[49]

---

[48] https://www.themix.net/tv-shows/bill-gates-ex-wife-melinda-slams-him-for-meeting-with-jeffrey-epstein-he-was-evil-personified/
[49] "The Lion the Witch and the Wardrobe" by CS Lewis is a uniquely symbolic and metaphoric story of the battle between good and evil.

And to our own selves be true!

Columbia U's Isaiah Sheffer stole my Joyce Festival, built an entirely new career on it.

There are many pejorative terms for alcoholics.

Those labels are applied without understanding or compassion. There should be far more for "Weinsteins."

However, the scary truth is that almost anything that can engage the human immune, digestive and endocrine systems too often and too regularly can create dependency – thence **addiction!**

The difference between a passion for, say, art, music, building, gardening, crafts, studying, knitting, sewing, cooking, entertaining and a million other pastimes, and *addiction*, is that anything done with Love creates, inspires, and enhances life and relations – and may also lead to professionalism and prosperity.

Addictions, however, lead to destruction, dissolution, depression, divorce, debt and dementia.

The most auspicious way of treating addiction, is with skilled Homeopathic treatment combined with a Twelve Step program.

Homeopathy clears the systems, and, in so doing, gradually removes the triggers for the desire of the addicting substance. During that process, the Twelve Step programs provide support, and companionship, but best of all, assist the addict to *keep the focus on the self and the appropriate actions and attitudes for the maintenance and survival of the afflicted person.*

Addiction is not a "weakness." Alcoholism is hereditary, i.e., genetic, seldom "acquired," and every drug addict of my professional acquaintance had an alcoholic parent or grand parent. Again, instead of criticising and condemning, be thankful if that is *not* in your heritage and commend the newly sober.

Ch30 - Ghoul School

"Ghoul school" refers to the corrupt branch of allopathy, not to the dedicated physicians hanging on by a thread against pressure to retire early.

In that context I am reluctant to pose possible strategies here, as the "ghoul school" will only misuse them, either purposely to "claim" and patent them at the behest of p-Harm-a, or to discredit Homeopathy, or indirectly, as we will not provide a "one size fits all" remedy for them to tamper with and proclaim as the latest "wunderkind" of the drugs and euthanasia industry.."

Only to ultimately abuse, discredit and "withdraw" from the market! After all, what's a few million in payouts to bereaved parents or spouses when TRILLIONS are safely lodged in a nice mountainy vault in Switzerland, etc...

Also, I *know* for a fact that NYS was collusive with the *harmaceutical industry in allowing its patients hospitalised in State Hospitals to be used for experimental purposes.

They took my patient who had been through hell and back, and was on his way to FULL RECOVERY, and they pressured him to undergo another procedure, that is, the implantation of a diaphragmatic pacemaker, which, in my professional opinion was completely unnecessary, and which set him back a few months.

Thanks to Homeopathy, he recovered relatively rapidly, did not need to return the Respiratory Unit and endured no further MRSA or other infections since my treatment.

This was a brilliant 76 year old gentleman who had been on "nil by mouth" for almost two years, fed by stoma, despite his ability to swallow his own saliva.

He obviously hadn't "suffered enough."

Unkindest cut of all, his brother was the Medical Director of a Hospital in Massachusetts, and convinced him that it was his duty as a priest, bishop and Christian to undergo that torture *for the good of others.*

*They could not bear the fact that I proved without a shadow of further doubt, that Homeopathy was light years ahead of ordinary *harma medicine, vastly superior in result, and most wonderful of all – without adding to the suffering of our patients!*

And still we trust them!

And sometimes I wonder if some patients *prefer* the *sturm und drang* of exchanging control of their own bodies for the attention in each "this will only hurt a bit" protocol. "Attention attention!" As they say in Hollywood!

As for "my body myself" and "no one controls my body" – what do misguided women expect when they allow ghouls in white coats to strip them, immobilise them and insert lethal instruments into their most protected areas in order to murder their babies????

Seriously... "no one's going to control me..." said every feminist pro-abort ever *walking into the abortuaries to give up total control of their bodies, their internal organs, the lives of their babies and their own life, death or survival!*

I mean, why be a fully developed, unique female, when you can be a pathetic form of "wannabe man!"

The AMA was established for the express purpose of eliminating Homeopathy from the face of the earth.

*harma docs could not compete with the survival and full recovery statistics from our Homeopathic Hospitals despite the egregious practice of dumping their worst patients on us. I dare them to match the results in the following chart:

CONFIRMED RESPONSES TO HOMEOPATHIC PROTOCOLS –
Practice of Deirdre McNamara, D. Hom

ASTHMA	Freedom from dependence on inhalers and steroids.	Multinational
ALLERGIES	100% complete cure where patient and family 100% co-operative.	Multinational
ANTHRAX	(Eschar) complete cure within 24 hours. (Natural - not lab Anthrax!)	NYC
CELLULITIS	100% cure – where antibiotics failed.	NYC
PTSD/Trauma	Full or significant recovery	Multinational
FRACTURES	Accelerated symphysis even with dx of osteoporosis.	Multinational
BURNS	Accelerated healing without scarring.	Multinational
Chemical Burn	Ocular - Accelerated healing within 24 hours after 72 hrs agony	NY
PNEUMONIA	Accelerated recoveries (Also Pleurisy, Bronchitis, "Covid," etc)	Multinational
PARALYSIS	Trauma: Restoration of sensation and mobility Thrombosis (stroke) Restoration of sensation and mobility	Multinational

PARKINSONS	Complete elimination of tremor, restoration of energy, mobility. Multinational
SEIZURES	Congenital, pediatric, severe, multiple, daily. 100% cure - one dose of correct remedy; one seizure following, none to date. UK (Telehealth)
INFERTILITY	100% success. No intrusive measures. Homeopathic similars administered. Babies then conceived naturally in US, India, Europe.
RESP UNIT	*Patient dependent on Respirator 24/7 x 16 months, weaned off Respirator within two months after continuous Homeopathic treatment. Transferred to assisted living unit for minimal assistance. Lived productive, active life for years until iatrogenic "mishap." I was not available – family funeral in Europe.*
"COVID"	100% full recovery rate within 24-72 hours. "Vaccinosis" Recovery within 24-72 hours.
POST SURGERY	*Three digits severed. Surgically restored, slow healing. Homeopathy restored sensation and motility within two weeks. Significant improvement end of week one.*
INFECTIONS	Hepatitis A, B, C fully cured within one to three weeks, tests completely free of viral load. Other infections, including one case of bacterial meningitis, etc. Multinational
COMA	Recovery within three hours. (Not officially recorded) NY (in hospital)

*Homeopathy was available on the UK NHS. US Health Insurance providers gave discounts to our patients - longer, healthier lives. They covered our treatments until "Hillary Health Care." Heads of State, "Royals"and Medical Directors consult us for themselves and families. Not allowed to refer patients, however. Saved NYS $1,000,000 per annum on just one patient. North and South Civil War combatants consulted our H forbears, faster recoveries. 97% **full recovery** in 1918 Flu epidemic, etc.*

Annotations

---

[i] Books of Kings (2 Kings 18:4; written c. 550 BC), the **Nehushtan** (/nəˈhʊʃtən/; Hebrew: נְחֻשְׁתָּן, romanized: *Nəḥuštān* [nəħuʃtaːn]) is the bronze image of a serpent on a pole. The image is described in the Book of Numbers, where Yahweh instructed Moses to erect it so that the Israelites who saw it would be cured and be protected from dying from the bites of the "fiery serpents", which Yahweh had sent to punish them for speaking against Him and Moses (Numbers 21:4–9).[i]

[ii] Dr Dermot Murray, GP, Knock.
[iii] "Befehl ist Befehl" ie "an order is an order" – the primary excuse at Nuremberg. "Operation Paperclip" was President Truman's "importation" to the USA of the worst of the Nazi collaborators.
[iv][v] Italics here indicate material added in May 2024

From: "The Real Anthony Fauci" email on April 14, 2023

In the United States, Covid jabs have led to more than 6,113 deaths, 5,172 permanent disabilities, 6,435 life-threatening events, and 51,558 emergency room visits.

All the while the government continues pushing mass vaccination… It is interesting that approximately half of the employees at NIH and the CDC **had been reported to not have received the injection**. (Author's note: In EU all politicians, diplomats, journos and doctors were exempt from travel restrictions)

This may sound outlandish, but give it a chance…

Utah State University's 2018 study from their Biological Engineering department, they have a study titled "Synthetic Snake Venom from the Coralotid Snake Phospholipase A2 by Genetic Engineering".

"Genetic engineering is the term. All they did was instruct E-coli bacteria how to make synthetic phospholipase A2 — snake venom — in bacteria!"

This is how they did it - V Factor Bio Weapon Genetic Engineering

In COVID-19 patients, they found multiple venom components that cause blood clotting and are called "pro coagulation activators" or Factor V Self-Clotters".

Tests confirmed that this Factor V can make blood clots all on its own!

Yes, you read that right.

When a person gets the jab, it damages red blood cells and makes them stick together, this is called **"sticky blood."**

Thrombosis of blood, or adhesive fibrins!

It's just crazy to see this study result…

In an Italian study, scientists confirmed 36 different venoms were present in those that had PCR tested positive for COVID.

PCR tests have been used for 20 years in venom research mRNA of snake venoms. They used PCR tests to identify all the different venoms that we're now finding in COVID-19 patients that are positive with a PCR test.

FACT: The PCR-negative test groups had NO VENOMS!

"Why are they using a PCR test which is 100% accurate in identifying the DNA, RNA, and mRNA of snake venoms if SARS-CoV-2 did not originate from venom?"

Venoms both natural or man-made (synthetic) are toxic and

dangerous.

That's why, we'd like to share with you this timely new e-book from Jonathan Otto:

CLOT SHOT: Sticky Blood & Chronic Diseases Caused by Deadly Spike Glycoproteins.

>>> *Download your FREE copy of CLOT SHOT: Sticky Blood & Chronic Diseases Caused by Deadly Spike Glycoproteins*

Inside Jonathan's latest eBook…

From
<https://mail.yahoo.com/d/folders/1?guce_referrer=aHR0cHM6Ly9sb2dpbi55YWhvby5jb20v&guce_referrer_sig=AQAAAHI0R8mRSICYSm2J6BtV7ozzfmI7IC-NaVAn5s54kGIvP3kmI6jYhsj0fA4fo1EP6pLbd8YuCv7CKG1fCYkeXnDVJmhhoLyyuHMCP5aWI5cOC1bkjQdPF3pTKEY5_RGM54Ft7tgefA7RyRhrmLKYln8mjwo5Z3t1saFeD_oxzaTJ>
iv

Note
"Ghoul school" refers to the corrupt branch of allopathy, not to the dedicated physicians hanging on by a thread against pressure to "amp up" the vax numbers or else retire early.

Dear Readers, I have done my best to counter the idiosyncracies of Microsofts' 10.5**

This program is so bad that I fear that the next one might be even worse.

Pre 2000 the "Word" programs were for writers. Now they are for pre – programmed bots. The level of complexity is distracting and a nightmare. One page has disappeared. Numeration adjusted.

I have reached the point, once again, of "publish or be d***ed!

My appreciation to all who look to content and not for pointscoring based on petty quibbles!

God bless you one and all,

Deirdre McNamara, Author.

About the author.

Deirdre Kelleher McNamara, D.Hom., made History as the first Homeopath to consult, *qua Homeopathic physician*, in any US Hospital in over a century.

Saving to the State of NY *per patient* was about $1,000,000 per annum. *One million dollars – **per patient!***

She was the first to warn about the mRNA bioweapon and her penultimate work, "Mitochondrial Murder" analyses the dynamics and risks of the "clotshot" and offers suggestions in limiting the lethality of the vile bioweapon. Nominated by *bookauthority.org* as one of the top ten books on RNA in 2024.

Prior to two attempts on her life by Cuomo's thugs, sabotage of her progress by the NIH, NYS, etc., she had a successful practice at TRS Professionals, in NY, Knock, Ireland and was Consultant to the sweet Missionaries of Charity and received the personal thanks of the late, great Saint Mother Teresa.

St Mother Teresa now has Homeopathic clinics all over Calcutta.

Despite the encouragement of the late Cardinal O'Connor and Mother Teresa, McNamara still finds a tension within her fellow Catholics, who tend to conflate Homeopathy with Herbalism or take a superstitious standpoint. Given the billions spent on suppressing the truth of our excellence – when practiced correctly – this is hardly surprising.

 "Homeopathy – Gift of a Gracious God" attempts to assure fellow Catholics of the consistency of our practice with the Commandments.

So far, Dr. D's survival rate in "CV19" patients is 100%.

Contact: drdhom@proton.me Tel: 215 558 5251 (Service)

Tangential but relevant: Dr. D's "Tribe of Cannibals: Operation Take

Down America" reveals a subversive arrangement between Columbia U, School of Sociology, George Soros, Koffee Annan, Obama and Holder to destroy Constitutional America – a 40 year experiment that failed horrendously, but then again, it was never for the benefit of the US Citizens and legal residents, at huge cost to the American Taxpayer.

Tragically, it's anomalies and "vices" are being unfolded across the USA, and, now, the world's gluttonous globalists, aided and abetted by their spurious spawn, the EU, and the Mid East homicidal Christophobes all collude in the destruction of the Christian world and what appears to be calculated, pre-meditated genocide by mass vaccinoses, abortion, abortifacient "birth control," mutilation of children, pornographic abuse of children, destroying their reproductive organs, their sweet souls and often even taking their lives. Add to that the DEI non binary –multi "gender" identity syndrome, and the rapid replacement of human intelligence by soulless pre- programmed robots.

[v] Page 66 – Fictional figures and possible Homeopathic solutions relative to their characters. For the serious student of Homeopathy, the remedies are put in random order. Have fun!
Pulsatilla, Natrum Mur, Platina, Sepia...

BOOKS BY DEIRDRE KELLEHER MCNAMARA
Contact: deirdresbooks@proton.me

LIST OF BOOKS AUTHORED BY DEIRDRE MCNAMARA, HOMEOPATHIST, AUTHOR, DRAMATIST, COMPOSER and CHOREOGRAPHER post 2000. Pre 2000, works are archived in US Library of Congress and National Library of Ireland.

Most are available from Amazon.com and online booksellers
MITOCHONDRIAL MURDER?
HOMEOPATHY IN THE TIME OF COVID
HEART OF MERCY
NEW CHRISTMAS STORIES FOR CHILDREN OF ALL AGES
A WHISPER OF ANGELS
CHRISTMAS NAUGHTY AND NICE *
SOS – For Survivors of Suicides
CHILD SEXUAL ABUSE – Never Call It Love
MEDITATIONS ON THE MYSTERIES OF THE ROSARY – A dramatist's view of Christ's life
THE DEMISE OF SENATOR DUFF – Fiction. Corrupt Irish politician meets a bitter end. Whodunnit? You decide!
THE TUSCANY EXPRESS – Use of Homeopathy in crises. 'Lite'
CELEBRITY CITY – Unexpected encounters with NY's celebrities.
IRISH GHOST STORIES
THE FAMINE REPORT – Irish Famine eye witness reports in dramatized form.
THE DISGUISE – Play on homelessness and drug addiction. Hopeful message. Written for use in fundraising. Easy, flexible design, and opportunity to "include" classes and groups...
NIC and CATULA – Abandoned kitten and sad little boy 'rescue' one another. 4th grade and above.

TOM and the HAPPY CAT – for very small, sick children.

IN PROGRESS: THE RISE OF SENATOR DUFF
IN RESCUE:
HIC EST QUIES MIEA;
HOMEOPATHY – GIFT OF A GRACIOUS GOD;

ARCHIVED:
SUMMER OF THE DISCONTENT; *
THE MAN IN THE MOON MADRIGOL; *
FUGUE ON AN AMERICAN THEME (Four parts) etc*

*Archived in the National Library of Ireland – cardboard box in
the basement?
Other works archived in the US Library of Congress

DRAMAS INCLUDE: "MERCY!"
 "IRISH GHOST STORIES: MISTLETOE, SWEET DREAMS, THE
HUNGER GRASS,"
 "NINe ELevEn,"
 "THE DISGUISE,"
"THE IRA MAN'S DAUGHTER,"
"A SOLDIER CAME KNOCKING,"
 "THE FAMINE REPORT,"
"AN EVENING WITH JAMES JOYCE AND FRIENDS," etc., etc…